PRIMARY HEALTH CARE AROUND THE WORLD

RECOMMENDATIONS FOR INTERNATIONAL POLICY AND DEVELOPMENT

About the Series

The WONCA Family Medicine series is a collection of books written by world-wide experts and practitioners of family medicine, in collaboration with The World Organization of Family Doctors (WONCA).

WONCA is a not-for-profit organization and was founded in 1972 by member organizations in 18 countries. It now has 118 Member Organizations in 131 countries and territories with membership of about 500,000 family doctors and more than 90 per cent of the world's population.

Primary Health Care Around the World
Recommendations for International Policy and Development
Chris van Weel, Amanda Howe

Family Practice in the Eastern Mediterranean Region
Universal Health Coverage and Quality Primary Care
Hassan Salah, Michael Kidd

Every Doctor
Healthier Doctors = Healthier Patients
Leanne Rowe, Michael Kidd

How To Do Primary Care Research
Felicity Goodyear-Smith, Bob Mash

Family Medicine
The Classic Papers
Michael Kidd, Iona Heath, Amanda Howe

International Perspectives on Primary Care Research
Felicity Goodyear-Smith, Bob Mash

The Contribution of Family Medicine to Improving Health Systems
A Guidebook from the World Organization of Family Doctors
Michael Kidd

Primary Health Care Around the World

RECOMMENDATIONS FOR INTERNATIONAL POLICY AND DEVELOPMENT

EDITED BY

Chris van Weel

Emeritus Professor of General Practice/Family Medicine
Radboud Institute of Health Sciences
Radboud University, Nijmegen, the Netherlands
Honorary Professor of Primary Health Care Research,
Australian National University
A Past President of WONCA

Amanda Howe

President of WONCA
Professor of Primary Care at the University of East Anglia
A Practising General Practitioner, UK

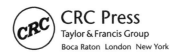

CRC Press
Taylor & Francis Group
Boca Raton London New York

CRC Press is an imprint of the
Taylor & Francis Group, an **informa** business

CRC Press
Taylor & Francis Group
6000 Broken Sound Parkway NW, Suite 300
Boca Raton, FL 33487-2742

© 2019 by Taylor & Francis Group, LLC
CRC Press is an imprint of Taylor & Francis Group, an Informa business

No claim to original U.S. Government works

Printed on acid-free paper

International Standard Book Number-13: 978-1-138-49867-9 (Paperback)
International Standard Book Number-13: 978-1-138-49868-6 (Hardback)

Visit the Taylor & Francis Web site at
http://www.taylorandfrancis.com

and the CRC Press Web site at
http://www.crcpress.com

Contents

Part IV   FROM DATA TO POLICY

Part V   CONCLUSIONS

Foreword

With the challenges of a global ageing population, to maintain maximum individual and population health throughout the lifespan and to deal with related social problems, a robust primary health care system is essential in every country. The Alma-Ata Declaration celebrates 40 years this year, and there will be a renewed statement that emphasizes the importance of effective primary health care to achieve universal health coverage.

Different countries around the world are developing and building their primary health care systems but with different characteristics according to culture, political will, health care financing and patient expectations. There are equity challenges for health care which include poverty, rurality and those in poor health. Key elements of effective equitable health care include accessibility and high quality, as well as availability and affordability. Culture and language also play a role.

There are a lot that countries and regions can learn from one another, and this book provides a lot of information on international policy and recommendations in developing primary health care from around the world. The reader will learn about the health care profile of various countries in the different regions around the world, collaborative health systems, implementation, transformation and improvement.

The World Health Organization (WHO) and all countries around the world recognize the value and importance of family medicine in primary health care. Family medicine is an essential component of primary health care, with practitioners or family doctors devoted to providing comprehensive continuous holistic care to individuals and families across all ages, genders, diseases and parts of the body. The practice of family medicine is the best assurance of quality and safe primary health care.

The authors have been leaders in family medicine, being President of the World Organization of Family Doctors (WONCA). WONCA represents over half a million family doctors in 150 countries and territories across the world. WONCA's mission is to improve the quality of life of people through fostering high standards of care in general practice/family medicine. Our members have a passionate interest and a key role to play in the delivery of effective and affordable personalized primary health care. The authors, Professor Chris van Weel and Professor Amanda

Howe, will share with us their experience and vision on primary health care gained during their work with WONCA and in their academic units over these years.

I am sure that those who, like myself, are devoted to advocating for the quality and safety of primary health care will enjoy reading this book and learning about primary health care system development around the world.

Donald Li
President 2018–2020
WONCA World Executive Council

Editors

Chris van Weel graduated from Leiden University in 1973 and practiced as a full-time GP in the Ommoord Community Health Centre in Rotterdam, the Netherlands, until 1985. In 1981, he obtained his PhD at the Erasmus University, Rotterdam, on a practice-based study of prevention.

In 1985, he was appointed professor of general practice at the Radboud University, Nijmegen, the Netherlands, and was head of the department from 1988 until his retirement in 2012. Since 2013, he has been affiliated with the Australian National University, as professor of primary health care research, currently in an honorary appointment.

From 2007 to 2010, he was president of the World Organization of Family Doctors (WONCA) after serving as chair of the WONCA Working Party on Research 1984–1998, and European president from 1998–2001.

His research focusses on primary care morbidity, multi-morbidity/co-morbidity and long-term outcome of chronic illness in family practice. The Nijmegen Academic Practice Network of the Continuous Morbidity Registration plays a central role in this research.

He founded the EU Erasmus programme 'Primary Health Care' that offers primary health care attachments and research electives to medical students from 15 countries.

He has been involved in CaRe since its founding in 1995, currently as a member of the Board of Governors.

Amanda Howe is a practicing family doctor, an academic professor and a national and international leader in family medicine. Since 2001, she has been Professor of Primary Care at the University of East Anglia, UK, where she was part of the founding team for a new medical programme. During her career, she has held multiple roles in undergraduate, postgraduate and faculty education, including being Course Director for the UEA medical programme during its early years of development and accreditation. She has particular expertise in the teaching and learning of professionalism and patient safety; in the models and effectiveness of involving family medicine in community-based medical education; and in resilience and doctors' wellbeing. She also has clinical research interests in primary care mental health, the contribution of patients to health care and in early interventions for risk factors. She served from 2009 to 2015 as an officer of the Royal College of General Practitioners, previously chairing their research committee and the UK Society for Academic Primary Care. She is president of the World Organization of Family Doctors (2016–2018). Her lifetime commitment is to making family medicine better – for patients, governments and for those doctors who choose to practice it!

PART I

INTRODUCTION

CHAPTER 1

A snapshot of primary health care around the world

Chris van Weel and Amanda Howe

Many countries in the world go through a transition of their health systems toward primary health care. In this, the care of patients is to be led from the community rather than the hospital, by a generalist rather than a specialist. This book presents a snapshot of this transition process: the current status of primary health care development around the world. It provides factual information, but even more on the tortuous journey of change. An essential feature of implementing primary health care is to apply generally valid principles under vastly different local conditions. This asks for concerted 'bottom-up' action under local conditions, and this makes the many experiences gained in the various countries equally valuable lessons for international collaboration. In three sections, it (1) addresses the importance of collecting information from the local health context; (2) presents an overview of information from studies in all regions of the world with respect to primary health care development; and (3) reflects on how findings on the status of primary health care can be used for policy development.

GENERAL POLICY OBJECTIVES

The World Health Organization (WHO) set the scene of this movement towards primary health care in 1978 with the Alma-Ata Declaration [1], which gained momentum when the impact of primary health care on health expenditure and population health became clear [2]. With the move of the place of care from hospital to community and from specialist to generalist, a number of perspectives are achieved.

Access and availability: Whenever people contact health care, it is usually in their local living environment: the community is where most people with most of their health problems are, most of the time [3]. It is also the best place to protect people against health threats and to support those with (chronic) health problems to preserve their functional capacity. This has been described as the 'ecology of health care' model [3], which illustrates the central position of community and living environment for the health of individuals. It emphasises the position of primary health care in its availability for unrestricted access for all health problems at the community level.

Responsiveness: The community base of primary care brings with it an involvement in that community and a focus on the prevailing social, cultural and economic conditions of that community as determinants of health [4]. From this context, primary health care is able to find the response to the most important health needs of individuals and populations over time [5,6].

Empowerment and resilience: From its community basis, primary health care integrates diagnostic and therapeutic interventions with prevention, health promotion and supportive care, helping individuals and communities to care for their own health as much as possible. This results in healthier, empowered individuals and more resilient communities [7,8].

Cost-effectiveness: Investment in primary health care is needed to realise these outcomes. But this investment will result in cost-effective health care due to savings and benefits elsewhere [7,9,10]. Through better population health at lower overall health care costs, primary health care provides strong support to affordable health care.

In summary, policy towards primary health care is able to achieve a number of objectives at the same time: financial, population health, resilience of communities. This may indicate the complex nature of primary health care, with its impact on individual and community – it may also indicate the complexity of this policy of change. It addresses the functioning of the health system, the performance of health professionals, the educational system of future professionals and, at the same time, the functioning of communities where people live. In other words, establishing a relationship with the local situation is paramount, and this implies a bottom-up approach to complement any centralized policy of health reform. The aim of this book is to support this bottom-up process.

The WHO, with its World Health Report of 2008 [11], has given a strong push for countries to pursue primary health care as the core of their health system. This got a further boost by the movement for universal health coverage [12], as part of the United Nations Sustainable Development Goals [13]: universal health coverage can only be realised when there are facilities – in the community – to access care; when the care provided is affordable; and when the investments in health care result in better population health. This is why primary health care should be at the core of any health system and these general policy objectives be realised.

PRIMARY HEALTH CARE AND FAMILY MEDICINE

The task of primary health care is to connect with the needs of populations and individuals coping with their health and disease, to function and perform. It asks for the competence to integrate prevention, cure and care, and to bring together the biological, psychological and social domains [14] while maintaining an engagement over time with individuals and populations [15]. This professional complexity asks for a multidisciplinary approach, of nurses, midwives, allied health professionals and family physicians [16]. Primary health care, in other words, is broader than family medicine, but there is no primary health care without family physicians.

FROM GENERIC PRINCIPLES TO THEIR IMPLEMENTATION IN THE LOCAL CONTEXT

The change of health care from the hospital to the community, from the specialist to the generalist is in itself a fundamental change – a change in the structure of the health care system, in the conditions and facilities under which professionals operate and engage patients, and in the training and education of health care professionals. Most, if not all, of this process of change is based on trial and error, and this book gives an insight into experience available: how the process of change takes shape under vastly different conditions, in rich and poor countries, countries with and without a tradition of social welfare and solidarity, with and without strong educational systems of physicians, nurses and other professionals. This 'natural variation' provides a richness in empirical experiences of how to succeed or fail, from which to learn and benefit.

Yet in this natural variation, a number of challenges are universal. Virtually everywhere in the world, medical specialists tend to dominate generalists, and physicians other health professionals. The management of diseases takes central stage over the support of individuals – in the functioning of the actual care, as well as in its academic support of teaching, training and research, and in the rules and regulations of the health system. These present universal challenges that have to be surmounted in implementing primary health care in local communities around the world. The experiences collected in this book should serve as a reference, and even more as an inspiration, for everyone involved in the development of community-based primary health care.

REFERENCES

1. World Health Organization (WHO). *Declaration of Alma-Ata 1978*. Retrieved from: www.who. int/publications/almaata_declaration_en.pdf (accessed May 1, 2017).
2. Starfield B. Is primary care essential? *Lancet* 1994; 344 (8930): 1129–1133.

3. Green LA, Fryer GE, Yawn BP, Lanier D, Dovey SM. The ecology of medical care revisited. *The N Engl J M* 2001; 344(26): 2021–2025.

4. World Health Organization (WHO). *Closing the gap in a generation*. Commission on Social Determinants of Health. 2008. Geneva, Switzerland.

5. Mezzich JE, Snaedal J, Weel C van, Botbol M, Salloum I. Introduction to person-centred medicine: From concepts to practice. *J Eval Clin Pract* 2011; 17: 330–332.

6. Maeseneer J de, Weel C van, Daeren L, Leyns C, Decat P, Boeckxstaens P, Avonts D, Willems S. From 'patient' to 'person' to 'people': The need for integrated, people-centred health care. *Int J Person Centred Medicine* 2012; 2(3): 601–614.

7. Starfield B, Shi L, Macinko J. Contribution of primary care to health systems and health. *The Milbank Quarterly* 2005; 83(3): 457–502.

8. Stange KC, Ferrer RL. The paradox of primary care. *Ann Fam Med* 2009; 7(4): 293–299.

9. Macinko J, Starfield B, Shi L. The contribution of primary care systems to health outcomes within Organization for Economic Cooperation and Development (OECD) countries, 1970–1998. *Health Serv Res* 2003; 38(3): 831–865.

10. Kringos D. *The strength of primary care in Europe*. 2012. (Thesis). University of Utrecht, the Netherlands. Retrieved from: www.nivel.nl/sites/default/files/bestanden/Proefschrift-Dionne-Kringos-The-strength-of-primary-care.pdf (accessed May 1, 2017).

11. World Health Organization (WHO). *The world health report 2008 – Primary health care (now more than ever)*. 2008. Geneva, Switzerland. Retrieved from: www.who.int/whr/2008/en/ (accessed May 1, 2017)

12. World Health Organization (WHO). Universal health hoverage. Retrieved from: http://www.who.int/universal_health_coverage/en/ (accessed May 1, 2017).

13. United Nations. Sustainable development goals. Retrieved from: http://www.un.org/sustainabledevelopment/sustainable-development-goals/ (accessed May 1, 2017).

14. Engel G. From biomedical to biopsychosocial. Being scientific in the human domain. *Psychosomatics* 1997; 38(6): 521–528.

15. Uijen AA, Schers HJ, Schellevis FG, van den Bosch WJ. How unique is continuity of care? A review of continuity and related concepts. *Fam Pract* 2012; 29(3): 264–71.

16. World Health Organization (WHO). Sixty-second World Health Assembly: Primary health care, including health system strengthening. 2009. Geneva, Switzerland: WHO. WHA62.12.

PART II

METHODS

International comparisons of primary health care policy: Experiences and methodology

Chris van Weel and Felicity Goodyear-Smith

The World Health Organization (WHO) Declaration of Alma-Ata [1] placed the development of primary health care on the health policy agenda, a development that gained further priority when evidence was presented of the contribution of primary health care to population health and containment of health costs [2, 3]. Since the end of the previous century, most countries in the world have been involved in reforms that aim to strengthen the responsiveness of their health system to the needs of their population and to reinforce the role in the community of family physicians, nurses midwives and allied health professionals. These reforms have generated experience in translating general principles of primary health care to prevailing local conditions [4], but they remain by and large 'experience-based': what was accomplished in one jurisdiction often remained unknown elsewhere, and might not be transferable to other settings. International comparisons can be helpful methods to clarify and appraise different experiences, using the natural variation under which primary health care is developed. This is further explored in Chapters 3 and 4.

AVAILABLE EXPERIENCES

In the past decade, detailed insight has been collected in the primary health care situation in Europe, North America, Australia and New Zealand [5–8]. In Europe, the fall of the Berlin Wall in 1989 led to a process of international collaboration to support the transition of former Eastern bloc countries into the European Union (EU), including health reforms and primary health care development. This culminated in two large European studies by the Netherlands Institute of Health Services Research (NIVEL) [7,8]. Chapter 8 presents some of these findings.

In North America, a conference, *International Learning on Increasing the Value and Effectiveness of Primary Care* (I LIVE PC) [5,6], brought together experts from seven countries to present common problems in primary care and share their experiential learnings. This approach had been piloted in 2010 [9] and formed the basis for in-depth discussions with policy makers to support the work on health reforms. Chapters 10 and 11 present some of these findings.

GENERATING MORE DATA

These resources provide a rich knowledge of understanding primary health care development in Western, developed countries. But for many countries or regions, data of the conditions under which health reforms have to be generated are scarce – see Chapter 3. To address this, the World Organization of Family Doctors (WONCA) Working Party on Research developed a user-friendly method to document primary health care around the world and stimulate dialogues of how the values of primary health care can be addressed within the constraints of different health systems [10]. Using a framework of 11 PowerPoint slides (Table 2.1), primary health care professionals should be able to present their country's situation addressing (1) country demographics; (2) the health system; (3) the role and position of primary health care; (4) the country's main health challenges; (5) the strengths and weaknesses of the system's ability to address the health needs of its population; and (6) lessons others could learn from their country.

With this method, comparisons of the implementation of primary health care policy have been made in virtually all regions of the world, with an emphasis on where primary health care implementation is most urgent: lower- and middle-income countries. Chapters 5, 6, 7, 9, 12 and 13 are based on this approach. The experiences reported in these chapters – usually performed without financial support – stress the relevance of international comparisons. At the same time, properly funded research will provide data with more depth, as comes forward in Chapter 8, based on EU-funded research. And this is a barrier: although international comparisons can provide important insights for primary health care development, research funding is often restricted to studies within national jurisdictions. In Chapter 3, possible avenues to cope with this problem are explored.

TABLE 2.1 Template for Presenting Countries' Primary Health Care Policy Implementation Status

Slide	Subject	Information to Be Presented
1	Country and presenter	Country, WONCA region, Presentation Meeting (place, date) Presenter and affiliation
2	Population demographics	Population size Map of the country Age and sex distribution Ethnicity, religion Unemployment rate Life expectancy
3	Structure of primary health care (PHC)	Proportion of health professionals working in PHC Ownership of practices Coverage of costs of PHC: health insurance, out of pocket
4	Disciplines working in PHC in the community	Disciplines constituting PHC (family physicians, nurses, midwives, allied health professionals) Availability of PHC disciplines and distribution in the country
5	PHC and integrated PHC teams	Role of PHC teams in provision of primary health care Describe types of practices and their proportion: • solo FP/GP, group practice, health centres Staffing of practices: • practice assistants, nurses, allied health professionals Access to support services (laboratory, radiology)
6	Community-based PHC	Proportion of PHC teams organised around a defined population Proportion of PHC teams with structural multidisciplinary collaboration vs. ad hoc structuring around individual patients' needs
7	Relation of PHC to other community services	Relation with social welfare, community leaders, patient representatives (formal, ad hoc – informal)
8	Impact of PHC on patient care	Evidence of the impact PHC has on patient care, population health, life expectancy, provision of services, overall costs
9	Benefits encountered	Factors supporting, enabling PHC development Summarise models of success • policy makers, academia, medical profession • PHC as part of teaching, training, education, research
10	Barriers encountered	Factors standing in the way of implementing community-based PHC • policy makers, academia, medical profession
11	Responsiveness to community needs	PHC's ability to focus on and respond to health needs of communities
12	Lessons for other countries	Summary of what works well and does not work well in PHC

For a template PowerPoint presentation that you can adapt directly to your requirements, please visit [http://www.globalfamilydoctor.com/plenarytemplate].

REFERENCES

1. World Health Organization (WHO). *Declaration of Alma-Ata 1978*. Retrieved from: www.who. int/publications/almaata_declaration_en.pdf (accessed May 1, 2017).
2. Starfield B. Is primary care essential? *Lancet* 1994; 344 (8930): 1129–1133.

3. Starfield B, Shi L, Macinko J. Contribution of primary care to health systems and health. *Milbank Quarterly* 2005; 83(3): 457–502.

4. Kidd M (editor). *The Contribution of Family Medicine to Improving Health Systems: A Guidebook from the World Organization of Family Doctors.* 2013. Radcliffe Publishing: London, UK. (2nd edition).

5. Phillips RL, Jr. International learning on increasing the value and effectiveness of primary care (I LIVE PC). *J Am Board Fam Med* 2012; 25(1): S2–5.

6. *J Am Board Fam Med* 2012; *25(1). Retrieved from:* http://www.jabfm.org/content/25/Suppl_1.toc (accessed 28 Jan 2016).

7. Kringos D. *The strength of primary care in Europe.* 2012. (Thesis) University of Utrecht, the Netherlands. Retrieved from: https://www.nivel.nl/sites/default/files/bestanden/Proefschrift-Dionne-Kringos-The-strength-of-primary-care.pdf (accessed January 28, 2016).

8. Schäfer WLA. *Primary care in 34 countries: Perspectives of general practitioners and their patients.* 2016. (Thesis) University of Utrecht, the Netherlands. Retrieved from: http://www.nivel.nl/sites/default/files/bestanden/w-schafer-pc34.pdf (accessed May 1, 2017).

9. Miedema B, Goodyear-Smith F, Gunn J, et al. Primary care: A comparison across five nations. *Can Med Assoc J Blog* 2015; (Parts 1–6).

10. WONCA. *WONCA research working party multi-national plenary panel project.* Retrieved from: http://www.globalfamilydoctor.com/site/DefaultSite/filesystem/documents/Groups/Research/WONCA%20Research%20Panel%20project.pdf (accessed January 28, 2016).

CHAPTER 3

International collaboration in innovating health systems

Chris van Weel, Deborah Turnbull, Emma Whitehead, Andrew Bazemore, Felicity Goodyear-Smith, Claire Jackson, Cindy L.K. Lam, Barbara A. van der Linden, David Meyers, Maria van den Muijsenbergh, Robert Phillips, Jose M. Ramirez-Aranda, Robyn Tamblyn and Evelyn van Weel-Baumgarten

Family Medicine Updates

From the North American Primary Care Research Group

Ann Fam Med 2015;13:86-87. doi: 10.1370/afm.1751.

INTERNATIONAL COLLABORATION IN INNOVATING HEALTH SYSTEMS

Aim and Background

Strong primary health care is critical to secure sustainable health care.[1] The *International Implementation Research Network in Primary Care* (IIRNPC) was founded to facilitate exchanges of experiences between countries in primary health care implementation.[2,3] Involvement of all stakeholders, and focus on local conditions to approach health problems in a broad social, economic, political and cultural context[1] are core components.

Based on these principles, a pre-conference was organized at the 2014 North American Primary Care Research Group (NAPCRG) conference to explore international aspects of innovating health systems to:

- Come to a better understanding of health systems, and their needs and potential for change
- Review models of success in changing health systems
- Analyze the role of research funding agencies in international comparisons to inform systems' change

A full report is available on NAPCRG's website at http://www.napcrg.org.

Methods and Findings

Health care systems from Mexico[5-7] and Hong Kong[8-10] served as case studies for critical appraisal, using the World Organization of Family Doctors (WONCA) instrument.[11] In both populations the available capacity of primary health care is limited, and policy makers are uncertain of health care consequences. Advocacy of primary health care policy and research were identified as a priorities for instigating and supporting change.

Three innovative international approaches were shared:

- The *Embassy Conversations* organized in Washington, DC, allowed policy makers to learn from health care reform in Australia, Denmark, and The Netherlands. Experts from these countries spoke in their US embassies so that they could be recognized as experts by their home governments. Clinical and policy reactors provided US and Canadian context.

- An Australian community-based team of family physicians and endocrinologists applied a co-creation approach, involving highest-need patients in their own health care, resulting in better outcome of diabetes care and risk reduction,[12] and lower hospitalizations,[13] with higher patient satisfaction and lower costs[14] compared with usual care.

- The EU *RESTORE* project addressed how improved communication with migrants in primary health care can overcome lingual and cultural challenges. Through Participatory Learning and Action, contemporary social theory methods,[15] and implementation of communication guidelines and training initiatives, the most vulnerable and difficult-to-reach populations were engaged.[16,17]

The shift to primary health care asks for a redirection of research towards the community setting. Four funding agencies: the US Agency for Healthcare Research and Quality (AHRQ),[18] the Australian Primary Health Care Research Institute (APHCRI),[19] the Canadian Institutes of Health Research (CIHR),[20,21] and the Netherlands Organization of Health Research and Development (ZonMw)[22,23] presented their approaches towards innovation and translation support.

All 4 commission funding to establish partnerships beyond the research community to other stakeholders, in order to guide change. Innovative approaches included trained implementation experts who serve as change agents.

Bi-national collaborative funding between APHCRI and CIHR[24] was highlighted, exploring the variation between countries as a natural research experiment. International comparison-of-care outcomes were seen as powerful support for health systems innovation and change, but funding agencies are often restricted in funding to their national jurisdictions. The most efficient way to obtain transnational comparisons is for researchers to collectively apply to their national agencies. Comparisons would benefit from a standardization of outcome measures.

Conclusions and Actions

On the basis of these findings, the IIRNPC decided to pursue the following next steps:

- Inform Mexican leaders about effective primary health care policy and implementation practices via a preconference at the 2015 NAPCRG annual meeting in Cancun, Mexico
- Review the systems of Japan, the Republic of South Korea, Hong Kong, Taiwan, and Singapore at a

workshop at the WONCA Asia Pacific Conference in 2015 in Taipei[11,25]

- The *Embassy Conversations* model will be promoted as a promising approach for engaging policy makers and lawmakers in health systems innovation
- Promote participatory research methodology as a meaningful tool for engagement with stakeholders
- Promote the value of international comparative outcome research for health systems' innovation:
  - The 4 funding agencies have committed to ongoing informal discussions to consider opportunities for collaboration over shared areas of interest
  - Pursue the development of a standardized set of primary health care-sensitive outcome measures.

Chris van Weel[1,2]; Deborah Turnbull[1,3]; Emma Whitehead[3]; Andrew Bazemore[4]; Felicity Goodyear-Smith[5]; Claire Jackson[6]; Cindy L. K. Lam[7]; Barbara A. van der Linden[8]; David Meyers[9]; Maria van den Muijsenbergh[1]; Robert Phillips[10]; Jose M. Ramirez-Aranda[11]; Robyn Tamblyn[12]; Evalyn van Weel-Baumgarten[1].

[1]Radboud University, Nijmegen, NL; [2]Auralian National University, Aus; [3]University of Adelaide, Aus; [4]Robert Graham Center, USA; [5]University of Auckland, NZ; [6]University of Queensland, Aus; [7]University of Hong Kong; [8]ZonMw, NL; [9]AHRQ, USA; [10]ABFM, USA; [11]Autonomous University of Nuevo Leon, Mexico; [12]CIHR; McGill University, Canada

References

For a complete list of reference, see https://www.napcrg.org/Conferences/AnnualMeeting.

Attribution

Weel C van, Turnbull D, Whitehead E, Bazemore A, Goodyear-Smith F, Jackson C, Lam CLK, Linden BA van der, Meyers D, Muijsenbergh M van den, Phillips R, Ramirez-Aranda JM, Tamblyn R, Weel-Baumgarten E van. International collaboration in innovating health systems. *Annals of Family Medicine* 2015;13:86–87. doi: 10.1370/afm.1751. Reproduced with permission.

CHAPTER 4

Variation matters and should be included in health care research for comparison of outcomes

*Chris van Weel, Robyn Tamblyn
and Deborah Turnbull*

Primary Health Care Research & Development 2017; **18**: 183–187
doi:10.1017/S1463423616000438

DEVELOPMENT

Variation matters and should be included in health care research for comparison of outcomes

Chris van Weel[1,2], **Robyn Tamblyn**[3] and **Deborah Turnbull**[4]

[1]Professor Primary Health Care Research, Department of Health Services Research and Policy, Australian National University, Canberra, Australia
[2]Emeritus Professor General Practice, Department of Primary and Community Care, Radboud University Medical Center, Nijmegen, The Netherlands
[3]James McGill Chair, Departments of Medicine and Epidemiology and Biostatistics, Scientific Director, Institute of Health Services and Policy Research, Canadian Institutes of Health Research (CIHR) and McGill University, Canada
[4]Chair in Psychology, University of Adelaide, Adelaide, Australia

Background: Health care is provided under the conditions in which people live and under the rules and regulations of a prevailing health system. As a consequence, 'local' circumstances are an important determinant of the actual care that can be provided and its effects on the health of individuals and populations. This plays in particular, but not exclusively, a role in community-based primary health care. Although this is generally accepted, there is little insight in the *impact* of the setting and context in which health care is provided on the outcome of care. **Aim:** This paper argues the case to use this natural variation within and between countries as an opportunity to be used as a form of natural experiment in health research. **Arguments:** We argue that analysing and comparing outcomes across settings, that is comparative outcomes of interventions that have been performed under different health care conditions will improve the understanding of how the real-life setting in which health care is provided – including the health system, the socio-economic circumstances and prevailing cultural values – do determine outcome of care. **Recommendations:** To facilitate comparison of research findings across health systems and different socio-economic and cultural contexts, we recommend a more detailed reporting of the conditions and circumstances under which health research has been performed. A set of core variables is proposed for studies in primary health care.

Key words: health systems; international collaboration; primary health care development; primary health care policy

*Received 8 March 2016; revised 3 September 2016; accepted 11 November 2016;
first published online 22 December 2016*

Rationale for context informing comparative outcome research to advance improvements in health systems and primary care

Most health problems are managed in the community, where a large majority of the population

are cared for, most of the time (Green *et al.*, 2001). As a consequence, local circumstances define the care that can be provided. This applies to the health system itself and its resources, as well as to the socio-economic circumstances and determinants of health (CSDH, 2008). Primary health care with its community base exemplifies the requirement for considering the context of care delivery and the variability it creates in the health status of the population it serves. Every setting is unique and its attributes need to be understood as a precondition for implementing quality care

Correspondence to: Professor Chris van Weel, Department of Health Services Research and Policy, Australian National University, 62 Mills Road, Acton, ACT 2601, Australia. Email: chris.vanweel@anu.edu.au

184   *Chris van Weel, Robyn Tamblyn, Deborah Turnbull*

(van Weel, 2007). What is true for primary health care is true for health care in general: that it is shaped by the circumstances in which it is provided. A strategy for diagnosis, prevention or treatment that is effective in one setting is not necessarily effective elsewhere (Siregar *et al.*, 2011).

Variation under which health care is provided is considered within some empirical paradigms as a research bias, which needs to be accounted for via study design and analysis. This paper argues the case to use this variation as an asset, to help to explain how seemingly similar interventions produce diverse outcomes. We argue that analysing and comparing outcomes across settings, that is comparative outcomes, allows us to understand the attributes of context, or real-life setting and conditions, that co-determine outcomes of care. Moreover, to advance scientific knowledge about the impact of context on variability in the quality and outcomes of care we specify a set of core variables that might be considered in conducting such research in primary care.

Understanding the attributes of the context and conditions in which health care is delivered, and the way this enhances or impedes its impact is important to further the effectiveness and quality of care. Comparisons of outcome of care between settings can be powerful in this regard. A recent example of the benefits of considering variability comes from a review of randomised trials conducted into health workers in sub-Saharan Africa, which identified nine contextual factors associated with performance (Blacklock *et al.*, 2016). International collaboration can support health systems to innovate and change (van Weel *et al.*, 2015). For example, pharma care coverage is a hot topic in many countries because all are challenged to produce optimal value for investment. The experience in Quebec was the first jurisdiction to institute mandatory universal prescription drug coverage through a public and private insurance approach, other regions and countries could learn from this experience through a comparison with their own performance: The Quebec policy reform showed a reversal of the international trend for poorer compliance in the most economically disadvantaged (Tamblyn *et al.*, 2014). Advancing the capacity to conduct international comparisons provides unique opportunities to examine the role of different health systems and policies on health outcomes and equity.

Primary Health Care Research & Development 2017; **18**: 183–187

It is important in this context to clarify and critically appraise the nature of outcomes that need to be considered in health systems and community-based primary care research. A good example is the 'paradox of primary care'; while subspecialists may achieve better disease-specific results, in comparison to generalists – primary care results in enhanced population health (Stange and Ferrer, 2009). Functional health status (Huber *et al.*, 2011) may be a more relevant outcome to inform primary health care and public health, than markers of disease while the latter will be pertinent to subspecialist interventions. Outcome selection will be justified by the study focus; specifically the impact of care on patients or populations, and/or the process or structure in which care is provided (Donabedian, 1988; 2005).

Implications and measuring quality

To compare outcomes of care asks for an analysis of the most important differences and similarities between settings. Understanding and interpreting variation are key features of comparative outcome research and this is at-odds with those paradigms of health research that aim to control the circumstances in which interventions are studied. Future research will continue to require the use of more sophisticated choice of designs that are appropriate for comparisons of complex interventions in different contexts, that will need to be informed by the views of multiple stakeholders including consumers and policy makers. Combining different domains and data sets (The National Centre for Geographic and Resource Analysis) is of great importance, while not all that matters may have been or can be, quantified. Capturing quantitative and qualitative data will enhance the understanding of differences between settings, requiring the use of use of matrices to combine mixed methods (Miles *et al.*, 1984). A substantial literature exists on alternative research paradigms for dealing with local context, both how to characterise it and how to modify trial design to measure its impact, founded in principles of realistic evaluation first developed about 20 years ago (Tilley and Pawson, 1997).

The quality of such research is marked by the richness of naturally available variation that can be included in the study of natural experiments,

Variation matters and should be included in health care research 185

enriched by the availability of substantial advancements in methodologies to control for potential biases in observational research. This is essential for research to support practice and move

Box 1 From efficacy to system redesign

Research paradigm	Questions addressed
Efficacy	Does this intervention work under controlled conditions?
Effectiveness	Does the intervention improve the health outcome of the patient when applied in everyday conditions?
Implementation	Can the intervention work when applied across settings?
System redesign	How to structure the system to facilitate relevant interventions?

from the creation of knowledge about what interventions *can* work to insight of their value of what works under different prevailing health care contexts that will allow us to optimise their effects. To achieve the expected advancement in the health of the population, we need to balance considerations and research investment to accelerate the transition from efficacy to effectiveness to implementation and to innovation in care (Box 1).

The issue: describing the context, especially in relation to primary care

Box 2 presents attributes that should be measured in assessing the context of care. To illustrate its application, a powerful example from two countries with highly comparable population health and socio-economic status, and also comparable level of medical education, is used as it shows the impact of an essentially different basis of financing general practice. This is especially notable in primary health care where professionals specialise *in-depth* in the patients' context, so as to be able to address the full *breadth* of their health problems. Comparing outcomes between primary health care studies therefore would benefit

Box 2 Antibiotics prescribed for respiratory conditions: Belgium and the Netherlands

Resistance to antibiotics is an important health problem that continues to increase and unnecessary prescribing is a major driver of this problem (Goossens *et al.*, 2005). There are marked differences between Belgium and the Netherlands in this respect, with much higher use in Belgium. Most prescriptions of antibiotics are initiated in primary health care, and in both countries evidence-based guidelines are available that promote restrained use of antibiotics (Belgian Antibiotic Policy Coordination Committee, 2008; Dutch College of General Practitioners, 2015).

The two countries are highly comparable in their population health status and socio-economic circumstances, and the main reason to explain the differences in prescriptions has to be found in the structure of the health care system. In the Netherlands patients are allocated to a family practice, receive all their health care through that practice with their family physician receiving capitation payment, Belgian patients are free to contact any family practice and family physicians are payed on the basis of discrete items for service delivered.

While the Dutch health care structure is relatively neutral to the actual content of care provided, in Belgium prescriptions play a role in securing practice income and binding patients to a practice. This may illustrate that insight into understand differences in prescribing and use of antibiotics depends on an understanding of the health system. A more restrained prescribing of antibiotics can be expected from a redesign of the Belgian health system.

186   *Chris van Weel, Robyn Tamblyn, Deborah Turnbull*

from a standardisation of how to describe the setting and context. To support comparative outcome studies we propose the development of a core set of primary health care sensitive measures.

Measuring the context of health care

A number of domains can be distinguished in the real-life world in which health care is provided, and which can be included in the reporting of studies to support policy makers and may facilitate the generation of hypotheses of 'context that matters':

* Health system
  Structure of health care towards access: navigated through primary health care versus patients'

freedom to access every physician; insurance and coverage (including that for mental health); availability of services; financial barriers for patients (co-payment, deductible); payment of provider (capitation, item for service, performance incentives); the contract relation between patient and provider: patients listing (rostered) with primary health care practices).
* Social welfare
  Pensions; unemployment benefits; sickness benefits; community support services for social needs.
* Population and society
  Population demographics (gender, age, social class, education and employment status, ethnicity, religious convictions, health status markers).

Box 3 Presentation of information on context of care

Domain	Item	Information	Presentation
Health system	Structure	Yes/no primary care based	Narrative
	Insurance	No/restricted/comprehensive	Narrative
	Financial barriers	Yes/no co-payment, deductable	Narrative, $
	Availability services	Waiting lists, shortages	Narrative, numbers/population
	Provider payment	Capitation/item for service/performance incentives	Narrative
	Patient's contractual relation with provider	Preferential provider/rostering-panels of patients/free access	Narrative
Social welfare	Pensions	Yes/no	Narrative
	Unemployment benefits	Yes/no	Narrative
	Sickness benefits	Yes/no	Narrative
	Community support services	Yes/no	Narrative
Population and society	Demographics	Age	Standard age classes
		Sex	F/M
		Social class	Standard class
		Education	
		Ethnicity	
		Religion	
	Population health	Life expectancy	
		Main causes of death	
		Dominant health problems	
Objectives of interventions	Diagnostic	Rule-in/rule-out/risk assessment	Narrative
	Therapeutic	Preventive/curative/palliative/functioning	Narrative

Variation matters and should be included in health care research   187

• Objectives of diagnosis and treatment
  A diagnostic intervention can aim to rule-in or rule-out a health problem or specify individual risk status. Treatment can have the objective to prevent a health problem, cure it, provide palliation and symptom relief or improve functional capacity.

Consistent reporting of the study context will ensure rigour in comparative outcome analysis and inform professionals, policy makers and service users how the context of care may enhance or impede outcome. A proposal to standardise descriptions is given in Box 3.

Conclusion

This paper has argued the case for comparative outcome research to support the development of (primary) health care interventions, the implementation of novel approaches and redesign of the health system. This requires the explicit and where possible standardised presentations of the context. Research methodology for comparative outcome studies is available, but its relevance is undervalued. Part of the problem is that national funding agents often restrict the use of their funds to their own national jurisdiction To overcome this problem innovations in the funding of health research are needed (van Weel *et al.*, 2015). First and foremost, though, is to understand the scientific and health benefits that can be realised by comparing the outcomes of health interventions across countries and jurisdictions. Routinely presenting information of studies' setting and context could help raising awareness of its importance and help generate more specific hypotheses for further in-depth research.

References

Belgian Antibiotic Policy Coordination Committee. 2016: Guideline: acute sore throat [Dutch]. BAPCOC. 2008. Retrieved 2 September 2016 from http://www.health. belgium.be/internet2Prd/groups/public/@public/@dg1/@acute care/documents/ie2divers/15616531.pdf

Blacklock, C., Gonçalves Bradley, D.C., Mickan, S., Willcox, M., Roberts, N., Bergström, A., and **Mant, D.** 2016: Impact of contextual factors on the effect of interventions to improve health worker performance in sub-Saharan Africa: review of randomised clinical trials. *PLoS One* 11, e0145206.

CSDH. 2008: Closing the gap in a generation: health equity through action on the social determinants of health. Final Report of the Commission on Social Determinants of Health. Geneva, World Health Organization. Retrieved 2 September 2016 from http://apps.who.int/iris/bitstream/ 10665/43943/1/9789241563703_eng.pdf

Donabedian, A. 1988: The quality of care: how can it be assessed? *Journal of the American Medical Association* 260, 1743–48.

Donabedian, A. 2005: Evaluating the quality of medical care. *The Milbank Quarterly* 83, 691–729.

Dutch College of General Practitioners (NHG). 2015: The Dutch College of General Practitioners (NHG) Practice Guideline Acute sore throat. Retrieved 2 September 2016 from https://www.nhg.org/standaarden/volledig/nhg-standaard-acute-keelpijn#Inleiding

Goossens, H., Ferech, M., Vander Stichele, R. and **Elseviers, M., ESAC Project Group.** 2005: Outpatient antibiotic use in Europe and association with resistance: a cross-national database study. *Lancet* 365, 579–87.

Green, L.A., Fryer, G.E., Yawn, B.P., Lanier, D. and **Dovey, S.M.** 2001: The ecology of medical care revisited. *The* New England Journal of Medicine 344, 2021–25.

Huber, M., Knottnerus, A.J., Green, L., *et al.* 2011: How should we define health? *British Medical Journal* 343, d4163.

Miles, M.B. and **Huberman, M.** 1984: Drawing valid meaning from qualitative data: toward a shared craft. *Educational Researcher* 13, 20–30.

National Centre for Geographic and Resource Analysis in Primary Health Care, the Australian Primary Health Care Research Institute. 2016: Access to maps, data, information & tools. Retrieved 2 September 2016 from http://graphc. aphcri.anu.edu.au/graphc_anu/graphc.html

Siregar, A.Y.M., Komarudin, D., Wisaksana, R., Crevel, R.v. and **Baltussen, R.** 2011: Costs and outcomes of VCT delivery models in the context of scaling up services in Indonesia. *Tropical Medicine and International Health* 16, 193–99.

Stange, K.C. and **Ferrer, R.L.** 2009: The paradox of primary care. *Annals of Family Medicine* 7, 293–99.

Tamblyn, R., Eguale, T., Huang, A., Winslade, N. and **Doran, P.** 2014: The incidence and determinants of primary nonadherence with prescribed medication in primary care: a cohort study. *Annals of Internal Medicine* 160, 441–50.

Tilley, N. and **Pawson, R.** 1997. *Realistic evaluation*. London: Sage.

Weel, C.v. 2007: Research in primary care: how to live-up to its needs? *Primary Health Care Research and Development* 8, 1–2.

Weel, C.v., Turnbull, D., Whitehead, E., Bazemore, A., Goodyear-Smith, F., Jackson, C., Lam, C.L.K., Linden, B.A. van der, Meyers, D., Muijsenbergh, M. van der, Phillips, R., Ramirez-Aranda, J.M., Tamblyn, R. and **Weel-Baumgarten, E. van.** International Collaboration in innovating health systems. *Ann Fam Med* 13, 86–87.

Primary Health Care Research & Development 2017; **18**: 183–187

Attribution

Weel C van, Tamblyn R, Turnbull D. Variation matters and should be included in health care research for comparison of outcomes. *Primary Health Care Research & Development* 2017;18:183–187. doi: 10.1017/S1463423616000438. Reproduced with permission.

PART III

REGIONAL PROFILES OF COUNTRIES OF THE WORLD

CHAPTER 5

Africa

Robert Mash, Akye Essuman, Riaz Ratansi, Felicity Goodyear-Smith, Klaus Von Pressentin, Zelra Malan, Marianne Van Lancker and Jan De Maeseneer

Page 1 of 6 Conference Report

African Primary Care Research: Current situation, priorities and capacity building

Authors:
Robert Mash[1]
Akye Essuman[2]
Riaz Ratansi[3]
Felicity Goodyear-Smith[4]
Klaus Von Pressentin[1]
Zelra Malan[1]
Marianne Van Lancker[5]
Jan De Maeseneer[5]

Affiliations:
[1]Division of Family Medicine and Primary Care, Stellenbosch University, South Africa

[2]Department of Community Medicine, University of Ghana, Ghana

[3]Department of Family Medicine, Aga Khan University, Tanzania

[4]Department of General Practice and Primary Health Care, University of Auckland, New Zealand

[5]Department of Family Medicine, University of Ghent, Belgium

Correspondence to:
Robert Mash

Email:
rm@sun.ac.za

Postal address:
PO Box 19063,
Tygerberg 7505,
South Africa

Dates:
Received: 07 Aug. 2014
Accepted: 07 Aug. 2014
Published: 05 Dec. 2014

How to cite this article:
Mash R, Essuman A, Ratansi R, et al. African Primary Care Research: Current situation, priorities and capacity building. Afr J Prm Health Care Fam Med. 2014;6(1), Art. #758, 6 pages. http://dx.doi.org/10.4102/phcfm.v6i1.758

Introduction

The Sixth PRIMAFAMED (Primary Health Care/Family Medicine Education Network) workshop on 'Capacity Building and Priorities in Primary Care Research' was held in Pretoria, South Africa (SA), from 22 to 24 June 2014. Delegates from the following countries attended the workshop: Ghana, Nigeria, Uganda, Kenya, Tanzania, Sudan, Malawi, Zimbabwe, Botswana, Namibia, SA, Zambia, Ethiopia, Rwanda, Mozambique, Swaziland, Belgium, and Denmark (Figure 1). Delegates were from established or emerging departments of family medicine and primary care in these countries. The central theme of the workshop was primary care research – the current situation, the priorities for research and the need for capacity building. This report gives a summary of the consensus on these matters that emerged from the workshop.

The motivation for the conference was derived in part from the involvement of Professor Bob Mash (SA) and Professor Olayinka Ayankogbe (Nigeria) in the World Organization of Family Doctors (WONCA) Global Working Party on Primary Care Research, which has a goal of promoting primary care research.

Process

A four-step process was followed leading up to this report on the final consensus:

1. Situational analysis: Each institution attending the workshop was requested to present a poster summarising their current research activities and output. The delegates reviewed these posters in an interactive poster session (Figure 2).
2. International perspective: Professor Felicity Goodyear-Smith addressed the conference on capacity building for primary care research (Figure 3) from her perspective as Head of Department of General Practice and Primary Health Care, University of Auckland; Founding Editor, Journal of Primary Health Care; Executive member, WONCA Working Party on Research; and Vice-Chair, International Committee, North American Primary Care Research Group.
3. Small group discussion: The delegates were divided into four groups to reflect on the situational analysis, give feedback on the current research priorities, define what capacity building was needed and give suggestions on how this capacity could be attained. Small groups were facilitated by Dr Akye Essuman (Ghana), Dr Riaz Ratansi (Tanzania), Prof Felicity Goodyear-Smith (New Zealand) and Prof Bob Mash (SA).
4. Consensus building plenary: Each of the four groups made a short Microsoft® Powerpoint presentation in plenary and these presentations were followed by a general discussion (Figure 4). The comments and additional reflections made during the final plenary were documented.

This report is a summary of the final consensus achieved through this process.

Situational analysis

The workshop considered the current strengths and weaknesses of primary care research in the African context from their perspective of the discipline of family medicine and primary care.

Strengths of current situation

The context of family medicine and primary care researchers

Family medicine and primary care is a generalist discipline which works in communities, primary care facilities and district hospitals. Little research currently takes place within this context and there is therefore a huge potential for almost any research to be useful and to make a difference.

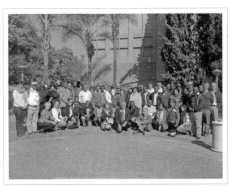

Source: Photo taken by authors
FIGURE 1: Delegates at the 6th PRIMAFAMED Workshop, 24 June 2014.

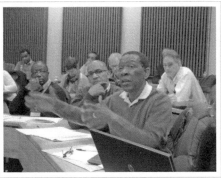

Source: Photo taken by authors
FIGURE 4: Final plenary discussion.

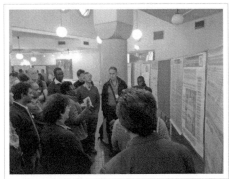

Source: Photo taken by authors
FIGURE 2: Delegates discuss the poster presentations.

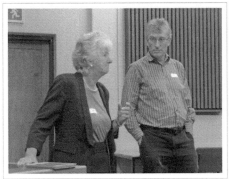

Source: Photo taken by authors
FIGURE 3: Professor Felicity Goodyear-Smith answers questions after her plenary address.

Understanding community health needs and strengthening primary healthcare are important aspects of any country's health system. Research performed in communities and primary care can be more relevant with regard to people's health and the translation of evidence into practice. The research agenda is more closely aligned with the needs of communities. For example, the community can be seen as a 'living laboratory' and community-oriented primary care can result in rich data derived from both homes and families. Because of its generalist nature, primary care touches on issues across the full burden of disease and tends to be more person-oriented – trying to make sense of how people see health and disease. There is a clear opportunity for a partnership between service, training and research within a culture of learning in communities and primary care. The African context will also provide unique opportunities for primary care research that are not found elsewhere. As exemplified by the participants of this workshop, there is both interest in and commitment to increase capacity and activity in the area of primary care research.

Support for research activities is increasing on a small scale

Many of the institutions represented are increasingly offering support for research activities and capacity building – for example through the Medical Education Partnership Initiative (MEPI). Some institutions are putting pressure on their staff to perform better in the area of research. Universities, of course, also receive substantial funding and, in some countries, subsidies for research activities and outputs.

The region does have some leadership and expertise to support research

It should be acknowledged that the region does indeed contain some of the research expertise required to both support and enable primary care research.

Training programmes require students to perform research

Currently, postgraduate training in family medicine at most institutions requires students to perform research as part of their training. In a few cases, the undergraduate programme also prepares people for research activities.

Opportunities exist for publication and presentation of research

Within the region there are a number of national, regional and international journals, such as the *SA Family Practice Journal*, the *East African Medical Journal* and the *African Journal of Primary Health Care and Family Medicine*. In addition, there are a number of opportunities to present at national and regional conferences such as the annual SA National Family Practitioners' Conference or the WONCA Regional Conference. Botswana is about to host its Second Family Medicine Conference.

There is an established culture of networking and collaboration

A number of networks and collaborations already exist in terms of developing training programmes through, for example, PRIMAFAMED and MEPI. There are also examples of research collaboration, such as with the Human Resources for Primary Care in Africa (HURAPRIM) project. This meeting itself demonstrated a huge potential for collaboration, not competition, between stakeholders. In some settings there may be opportunities for collaboration between the private and public sector.

There is an opportunity for interdisciplinary research teams

As the clinical nature of family medicine and primary care is to work in teams of community health workers, nurses, mid-level health workers, doctors and allied health professionals, there is an established culture of cooperation. This has the potential to enable interdisciplinary research approaches.

Weaknesses in the current situation

Some delegates preferred to re-frame weaknesses as challenges and opportunities for future development.

Low research capability

Departments of family medicine and primary care have few academic staff and those that do exist often lack expertise in performing and supervising research. Most staff are either newly qualified or relatively junior and many postgraduate research projects are designed poorly or lack social and scientific value. Most research performed is descriptive and small scale and there is a lack of capacity to perform more experimental and analytical types of research on a larger scale.

Low research capacity – people, funding and resources

Large-scale funding is mostly from overseas donors and funding agencies and is not targeted at strengthening primary healthcare outside of certain priority diseases such as HIV and tuberculosis (TB). On the other hand, the lack of capability amongst researchers makes it difficult for them to compete for and obtain large-scale international funding; researchers may also fail to be aware of or take advantage of the smaller-scale grants and funding opportunities available locally. At this time, researchers should focus on low-cost, high-impact projects.

Some countries reported that they still have limited or unreliable access to the internet and key software and that their institutions could not afford access to many journals.

The demands of clinical service and teaching reduce the available time and energy for a focus on research. In addition, the number of postgraduate students at a Masters level to help drive research is also small in many countries.

Failure to publish and disseminate research findings

Despite the opportunities listed above, much of the research performed is not submitted for publication or presented at conferences. Research, however, should be judged not so much by the impact factor of the journal as by its impact on policy and practice, which may depend on strategies other than just publication.

High inertia in the system

The process of obtaining ethical approval and permission to perform research is a long and bureaucratic process in many institutions. This may be compounded by a lack of support for the types of research performed most commonly in primary care, for example qualitative and action research-type projects. Review committees and boards do not usually have representatives from the family medicine and primary care context.

Lack of innovation in types of research

People working in primary care may not see the rich opportunities for research that are a part of their daily work because of their prior exposure to types of research performed in referral hospitals, laboratories and clinical trials – which become normative in terms of their understanding of what research should be like. The opportunities for evaluation of community health needs, surveys, quality improvement studies, programme evaluation, participatory action and qualitative research are lost.

Poor coordination of research activities

Researchers often work on small-scale projects in isolation and without alignment to a clear set of local priorities. Few departments have a clearly agreed-upon research agenda.

Lack of collaboration in research activities

Despite the existing collaboration on training, there is relatively little collaboration between institutions and countries on primary care research projects. There is also a lack of awareness of the expertise and support that could be obtained from researchers within the same institutions, but from different disciplines. For example, there is no database of established researchers in the field and potential mentors.

Lack of support from academic and government policymakers

The relatively low status of family medicine and primary care in most universities and the hospital-centric view of many health systems, means that there is a relative lack of understanding and support from key leaders and stakeholders for primary care research. There is often no national plan or strategy for primary care research. On the other hand, researchers may also lack insight into the national research priorities that have been identified.

Future priorities in primary care research

The delegates recognised that it is not possible to set specific priorities for the whole of Africa and that each country and institution must set its own such priorities for the local context. Nevertheless, some general comments and pointers were made based on the typology of primary care research suggested by John Beasley and Barbara Starfield.

General comments

Primary care research should shift the focus from hospitals to primary healthcare and communities. Research should have clear social value to communities and scientific value to decision makers. In addition, research should use a mix of different methods and range across the whole of the typology outlined below.

Basic research

This should focus on the adaptation (e.g. of the primary care assessment tool) or development (e.g. family physician impact assessment tool) of key tools for use in primary care research in the African context.

Clinical research

Most research is currently in this domain. Research should focus across the whole local burden of disease (e.g. HIV/AIDS, TB, non-communicable chronic diseases, injury and violence, maternal and child mortality, etc.) and look at cost-effective interventions in order to improve the quality of care or community-oriented primary care.

Health services

There is currently little research looking at the core dimensions of effective primary healthcare – access, continuity, coordination, comprehensiveness and efficiency. This, however, should be a priority area in terms of strengthening the primary healthcare system. Strengthening the health information system within the district is also a priority.

Health systems

Most research at this level has been on the contribution of family medicine, family physicians and primary care doctors to the health system. As this is still a contested issue in most African countries, this remains a priority – evidence for the contribution of family medicine and how family physicians should be utilised within the district health system. A broader theme is that of research on the human resources for primary healthcare in the African context.

Educational research

As family medicine and primary care training programmes are in a state of design and development in many countries, the need for supportive research to guide this process remains a priority. For example, curriculum development and faculty development are key topics.

How to build capacity for primary care research

The development of both capability and capacity were seen as being a maturation process over time and not just an issue of training. Given the rich primary care context and the growing number of role players, the building of their capacity may unlock a new stream of research activity.

Contribution of regional and international networks in family medicine and primary care

South-South collaboration, as well as North-South, should be enabled by the existing networks such as PRIMAFAMED, WONCA and MEPI. These networks should enable the sharing of expertise, resources and tools for research, as well as published research from within the network. They could also be a way of sharing information on funding opportunities and grants. These networks should also encourage the emergence of joint projects and provide training opportunities. Mentors and mentees should be connected and a database of expertise and mentorship created. Regional meetings are an opportunity for networking, benchmarking between countries, training and strategic planning. Websites or list servers operated by these networks can be a means of disseminating information and resources and should also become more interactive. Those better off in terms of resources should take the lead and involve others.

Contribution of the individual countries and academic institutions

Develop national policy which includes a focus on primary care research

Enable funding mechanisms for emerging primary care researchers. The subsidy scheme in SA by the Department of Education to universities linked to research outputs is a useful incentive and funding mechanism.

Universities should look at building formal links for primary care research

Universities and faculties should look at how orientation to and preparation for research is built into the undergraduate programmes (e.g. research toolbox, extra credit for research). Developing skills in evidence-based practice can complement the development of research capability. They should also create opportunities for the presentation and even in-house publication of research, with incentives and prizes for participation, thus encourage emerging researchers. In addition, universities and faculties should ensure that the process for ethics approval and permission to perform research is an efficient process that supports primary care research.

Accepting the research assignment for the MMed in the format of a journal article and incentivising publication as an option for assessment during the degree (i.e., do not need external examination if accepted for publication through peer review by an accredited journal) can be a further means of encouraging throughput and publication.

Contribution of the departments of family medicine and primary care

Each department should develop a clear research agenda and strategy for capacity building, which can give direction to staff and students in terms of their research questions and topics. This should also be communicated to the broader faculty. It is important to ensure that student projects are aligned with this agenda and bring multiple small-scale individual projects together to make a larger, more integrated whole.

Departments should engage with the communities served when setting the research agenda as this will ensure more social accountability. In addition, they should collaborate with local research expertise (e.g. public health) in order to deliver on the research agenda set above. The possibility of interdisciplinary research teams should be explored, which would also encourage critical thinking from different perspectives.

Partnership with health services and policy makers would ensure that research is relevant and that findings will be incorporated into decision making.

It is essential to develop a research culture – reward and celebrate research outputs and link more experienced researchers with emerging researchers. In this way, it will be possible to integrate service, learning and research – *research what you do*.

Departments and researchers should make use of resources such as the 10 articles just published on primary care research methods in the *African Journal of Primary Health Care and Family Medicine*. In addition, they should ensure that they have registered with the journal and get e-alerts of published articles.

As well as making full use of local opportunities for training and funding, it would be worth considering having a designated primary care research champion who can link with others in the region and meet at WONCA or PRIMAFAMED.

Training issues

Training needs can be met at all levels, for example, distance learning courses from the broader international community, training during PRIMAFAMED or WONCA meetings in the region, by the University or Faculty, or even within the specific department:

- Create opportunities for advanced research training through doctoral degree programmes. Aim for each department to have at least one person with a PhD who is able to supervise and capacitate others. Look for funds to support this initiative, capacity for doctoral supervision and opportunities for training (e.g. Stellenbosch University African Doctoral Academy).
- Provide courses or retreats on scientific writing skills for proposals, grants, reports and publications.
- Provide courses on relevant methodologies for primary care researchers.

Conclusion

This conference provided an opportunity for key role players from academic departments of family medicine and primary care in Africa to interact on the topic of building capacity for primary care research. Delegates collaborated on a situational analysis, discussed the current priorities and considered ways of building more capacity in the African context.

Acknowledgements

The authors wish to acknowledge the participation of the following people in the conference:

Abdelnasir Mohammed (Sudan), Abraham Guyse (Nigeria), Andrew Ross (South Africa), Antony Mutara (Zimbabwe), Assegid Tucho (Ethiopia), Ayoade Adedokun (Nigeria), Billy Tsima (Botswana), Carien Lion-Cachet (South Africa), Daniel Ashebir (Ethiopia), Elsie Kigulie-Malwadde, Evans Chinkoyo (Zambia), Festo Njuki (Uganda), Francis Auiman (Swaziland), Gehrard Kweku Ofori-Amankwah (Ghana), Graham Bresick (South Africa), Honey Mabuza (South Africa), Indiran Govender (South Africa), Innocent Besigye (Uganda), Jannie Hugo (South Africa), Jimmy Chandia (South Africa), Jude Tadeo Onyango (Uganda), Kalay Moodley (South Africa), Kathryn Spangenberg Craig (Ghana), Longin Barongo (Namibia), Louis Jenkins (South Africa), Luckson Dullie (Malawi) Maaike Flinkenflögel (Rwanda), Marcus Goraseb (Namibia), Marietjie de Villiers (South Africa), Martha Makwero (Malawi), Mergen Naidoo (South Africa), Michelle Torlutter (South Africa), Mpundu Makasa (Zambia), Muriel Falalla (Zimbabwe), Mustafa Khoghali (Sudan), Nathaniel Mofolo (South Africa), Nazlie Beckett (South Africa), Ndifreke Udonwa (Nigeria), Nthabi Phaladze (Botswana), Ntokozo Dladla (South Arica), Parimalarani Yogeswaran (South Africa), Patrick Chege (Kenya), Per Kallestrup (Denmark), Peter Kirabira (Uganda), Riaz Ratansi (Tanzania) Sameh Mohamed Talab Aiash (Egypt), Shabir Moosa (South Africa), Shehnaz Munshi (South Africa), Stephen Reid (South Africa), Stephen Pentz (South Africa), Sunanda Ray (Zimbabwe), Teddy Nagaddya (Uganda), Titus Kahiga (Kenya) Vincent Setlhare (Botswana), Vincent Cubaka (Rwanda), Vincent Mubangizi (Uganda), Walaa Ali (Sudan), Werner Viljoen (South Africa), Wim Peersman (Belgium).

Funding

The workshop was funded by grants received from the European Union (SA), Medical Research Council (SA), SURMEPI (SA) and INCO (Belgium).

Stellenbosch University Rural Medical Education Partnership Initiative is supported by the U.S. President's Emergency Plan for AIDS Relief through the Health Resources and Services Administration (HRSA) under the terms of T84HA21652. This workshop has been conducted with the financial assistance of the European Union. The contents of this document are the sole responsibility of the authors and can under no circumstances be regarded as reflecting the position of the European Union.

Competing interests

The authors declare that they have no financial or personal relationship(s) that may have inappropriately influenced them in writing this article.

Authors' contributions

R.M. (Stellenbosch University) facilitated the whole process, one of the small group discussions and prepared the manuscript. A.E. (University of Ghana) and R.R. (Aga Khan University) each facilitated and summarised a small group discussion and approved the final manuscript. F.G-S. (University of Auckland) facilitated and summarised a small group discussion, provided the keynote address and approved the final manuscript. K.V.P. (Stellenbosch University) recorded and summarised the final consensus and approved the final manuscript. Z.M. (Stellenbosch University) recorded and summarised the final consensus and approved the final manuscript. M.V.L. (University of Ghent) coordinated the conference and poster presentations and approved the final manuscript. J.D.M. (University of Ghent) facilitated and summarised the situational analysis and approved the final manuscript.

Attribution

Mash R, Essuman A, Ratansi R, Goodyear-Smith F, Von Pressentin K, Malan Z, Van Lancker M, De Maeseneer J. African primary care research: Current situation, priorities and capacity building. *African Journal of Primary Health Care & Family Medicine* 2014;6(1):Art. #758. http://dx.doi.org/10.4102/phcfm.v6i1.758. Reproduced with permission.

CHAPTER 6

Asia-Pacific

Chris van Weel, Ryuki Kassai, Gene W.W. Tsoi, Shinn-Jang Hwang, Kyunghee Cho, Samual Y.S. Wong, Chong Phui-Nah, Sunfang Jiang, Masako Ii and Felicity Goodyear-Smith

Debate & Analysis

Evolving health policy for primary care in the Asia Pacific region

Most countries experience major challenges to their health systems. The factors behind this global trend are increasing health costs and diminished returns on healthcare investment for ageing populations. Where the primary healthcare function is formally structured in the health system, and professionals are educated for their specific tasks, the performance of the system is improved: better primary health care leads to better population health at lower healthcare costs.[1] This makes strengthening primary health care a global strategy to secure sustainable care.[2] The value of international collaboration in implementing primary healthcare policy was exemplified by the I LIVE PC conference in 2011 in Washington.[3] A critical feature of this is the modification and adaptation of general principles to the prevailing local conditions: primary health care must be built up from the community level where it has to operate.[4] For this, a good understanding of the existing health system is important in initiating reforms. There is growing insight in primary health care in Europe and North America,[3,5] but data are scarce for many countries or regions.[6] To address this, the World Organization of Family Doctors (WONCA) took the initiative to document how primary care is organised around the world, and created dialogues on how the values of primary care can be addressed within the constraints of different healthcare systems.[6] A plenary symposium at the 2015 WONCA Asia Pacific regional conference in Taipei, Taiwan, offered an opportunity to compare the health systems of six member organisations of WONCA — China (Shanghai region), China (Hong Kong), Japan, Republic of Korea (South Korea), Singapore, and Taiwan — and document their experiences in the implementation of policy. The six presentations were structured on the format and method developed by the WONCA Working Party on Research.[6] The discussions that followed focused on five aspects of policy implementation: the strengths and weakness of each system; priorities for change; the available capacity in the system to address and process major changes; setting-specific and joint Asia Pacific regional needs to support this process of change; and priorities in international collaboration to support change.

China — Shanghai

Healthcare reform in Shanghai is driven by a floating and increasingly ageing population.[7] There is poor referral between primary, secondary, and tertiary care, resulting in disordered medical consultations. The current challenges include how to provide high-quality primary care. More than 200 community health centres have been set up; the priorities for change include improving the quality and quantity of primary healthcare providers and establishing effective two-way referral systems. A healthcare system oriented to primary care should be implemented by government reform.

China — Hong Kong

Although Hong Kong has some of the best public health outcomes in the world, there is poor integration between primary and secondary care, as well as between private and public care, resulting in duplication of resources and doctor-shopping. Within primary care, the current challenges include differing standards of care provision and fragmented primary care.[8] The priorities for change include realigning the hospital-oriented healthcare system to a patient-focused healthcare system centred on primary care. This will require the government to put primary care at the centre of health system reform.

Japan

Despite having universal health insurance coverage since 1961, Japan is an example of a society that is underserved by an ill-defined primary care system with fragmentation and hospital centralism.[9] Faced with a rapidly ageing population and growing social security expenditures, Japan needs major reforms to reduce waste and enhance cost-effectiveness. A national system to accredit training programmes, including for general practice, has finally been introduced. A nationwide database project with international collaboration has been initiated to prospectively show the content and quality of general practice, to be ensured by standardised professional development.

"This lack of integration led to duplicated care, overuse of facilities, and wasting of precious resources that threatened the sustainability of the health system."

Republic of Korea

Healthcare coverage in South Korea consists of National Health Insurance and Medical Aid. There is a very weak gatekeeper system, and fee-for-service is the main payment method. The easy accessibility to any specialty and the low medical costs are major benefits for patients. Over-consumption and excessively high frequency of specialist consultation are major problems for the medical system.[10] The government and the primary care group seek to strengthen primary care but this is opposed by the medical society governed by the specialist group.

Singapore

Ranked by Bloomberg as the most efficient healthcare system in the world in 2014, Singapore's system has primary care as its foundation. However, not having a fixed primary care doctor and doctor-shopping have resulted in fragmented patient care. With an ageing population and an increased chronic disease burden,[11] priorities for change include patient 'empanelment' to clinical practices and teams of healthcare professionals, new care delivery, and payment models that better support chronic disease management. The government's continued support for greater collaboration between public and private primary care clinics[12] is imperative to ensure sharing of limited resources.

Taiwan

Taiwan's National Health Insurance has a high coverage rate, easy access, and high patient satisfaction, and it provides consistent healthcare quality. The current challenges include frequent ambulatory care visits and medical resources being wasted because of no strict referral system and only limited financial incentives for patients to choose primary care visits.[13] The priorities for change include improving the quality of primary care and shifting from hospital-oriented health care to community primary care. Integrated primary care, including a family doctor

"To secure access to high-quality health care for all, every health system will have to provide strong primary health care as its basis. Learning from others ... through ... sharing of experiences ... will ... support this."

programme (community medical group), has been initiated to solve these problems.

The presentations referred to many problems and uncertainties encountered when improving local health systems. This came forward in particular in the experiences in mainland China, where the recent decision to promote primary health care highlighted the need to build the family medicine workforce more or less from scratch. WONCA's mission has for long been to help countries build primary care and family medicine leadership in their local context through the establishment of national colleges and academies of family physicians.[14] It currently, has member organisations in 131 countries (http://www.globalfamilydoctor.com/).

Referred to at the same time was a next phase in primary care development. Their experiences were based on strong societal and economic development, with substantial improvements in population health and in general high levels of (technical) health care for populations covered by health insurance. From here, the challenges were not only in changing existing structures but also building where there had been nothing before.

An emphasis on provider-driven (instrumental) interventions led to poor integration between professionals. Where there was integration this was vertical,[14] leading to stand-alone disease-centred care. This lack of integration led to duplicated care, over-use of facilities, and wasting of precious resources that threatened the sustainability of the health system. A common feature was the absence of a primary healthcare function in the system to coordinate and horizontally integrate the care provision towards the needs and priorities of individuals and communities. With no restrictions to practise in the community, every specialist can claim 'primary health care'. This leads to variation in the quality of care and makes a primary healthcare function in the health system a priority. For primary health care to be able to lead, it is essential to introduce professional training in primary health care — including in family medicine — as the mandatory condition to practise in the community.

To move to primary health care, stakeholders near to policymakers, notably patients and community leaders, must work in a relation of trust with family physicians and other primary healthcare professionals. Shanghai and Singapore's community-based structure of health care is strong, and could be reinforced by introducing 'panels': individuals registered with a family practice to contract all their health care. Most countries could learn from how both Singapore and Hong Kong have built on their SARS experiences by creating facilities in polyclinics and community health centres to assess at-risk patients in isolation.

The workshop highlighted the need for better integration of care between different providers as well as with social services. Many countries share this need and this may emphasise the importance of horizontal integration based on a generalist primary care function.[15] This is directly related to the second need the workshop highlighted. To deliver its potential the generalist primary care function has to be built on competent professionals. Strengthening the primary care workforce through education and training directed at the core values of primary care[14] is again an issue for many countries. The workshop brought together in a pragmatic way experiences of only six WONCA member organisations and a more comprehensive review, including countries from other regions, may have presented other needs and priorities. This should therefore encourage a further international collaboration to review the implementation of primary healthcare policy. To secure access to high-quality health care for all, *every* health system will have to provide strong primary health care as its basis. Learning from others in implementing primary healthcare policy through international sharing of experiences — their challenges, failures, and successes — will continue to support this.

Chris van Weel,
Emeritus Professor of General Practice, Department of Primary and Community Care, Radboud University Medical Center, Nijmegen, the Netherlands; Honorary Professor of Primary Health Care Research, Department of Health Systems Research and Policy, Australian National University, Canberra, Australia.

ADDRESS FOR CORRESPONDENCE

Chris van Weel
Department of Primary and Community Care, Radboud University Medical Center, 117 ELG, PO Box 9101, 6500HB Nijmegen, the Netherlands.
**E-mail: chris.vanweel@radboudumc.nl
chris.vanweel@anu.edu.au**

Ryuki Kassai,
Professor of Family Medicine/General Practice, Department of Community and Family Medicine, Fukushima Medical University, Fukushima, Japan.

Gene WW Tsoi,
Family Physician and Past President and Council Member, Hong Kong College of Family Physicians, Hong Kong.

Shinn-Jang Hwang,
Vice Superintendent, Taipei Veterans General Hospital; Professor of Family Medicine, National Yang-Ming University School of Medicine, Taipei, Taiwan.

Kyunghee Cho,
Professor of Family Medicine, Department of Family Medicine, NHIMC Ilsan Hospital, Korea.

Samuel YS Wong,
Professor of Family Medicine and Primary Health Care, Division of Family Medicine and Primary Healthcare, School of Public Health and Primary Care, Chinese University of Hong Kong, Hong Kong.

Chong Phui-Nah,
Chief Executive Officer, Adjunct Associate Professor, Family Physician, Senior Consultant, National Healthcare Group Polyclinics, Singapore.

Sunfang Jiang,
Professor of General Practice, Department of General Practice, Zhongshan Hospital Fudan University, Shanghai Medical School Fudan University, China.

Masako Ii,
Professor of Health Economics, School of International and Public Policy, Hitotsubashi University, Tokyo, Japan.

Felicity Goodyear-Smith,
Professor of General Practice, Department of General Practice and Primary Health Care, University of Auckland, Auckland, New Zealand.

Provenance
Freely submitted; not externally peer reviewed.

Competing interests
The authors ha declared no competing interests.

©**British Journal of General Practice**
This is the full-length article (published online 27 May 2016) of an abridged version published in print. Cite this article as: **Br J Gen Pract 2016;
DOI: 10.3399/bjgp16X685513**

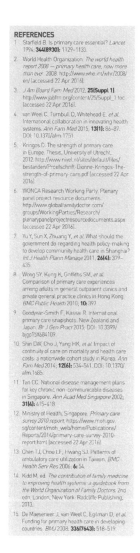

REFERENCES

1. Starfield B. Is primary care essential? *Lancet* 1994; **34(8930):** 1129–1133.

2. World Health Organization. *The world health report 2008 — primary health care, now more than ever.* 2008. http://www.who.int/whr/2008/en/ (accessed 22 Apr 2016).

3. *J Am Board Fam Med* 2012; **25(Suppl 1)**. http://www.jabfm.org/content/25/Suppl_1.toc (accessed 22 Apr 2016).

4. van Weel C, Turnbull D, Whitehead E, *et al.* International collaboration in innovating health systems. *Ann Fam Med* 2015; **13(1):** 86–87. DOI: 10.1370/afm.1751.

5. Kringos D. The strength of primary care in Europe. Thesis, University of Utrecht, 2012. http://www.nivel.nl/sites/default/files/bestanden/Proefschrift-Dionne-Kringos-The-strength-of-primary-care.pdf (accessed 22 Apr 2016).

6. WONCA Research Working Party. Plenary panel project resource documents. http://www.globalfamilydoctor.com/groups/WorkingParties/Research/plenarypanelprojectresourcedocuments.aspx (accessed 22 Apr 2016).

7. Yu Y, Sun X, Zhuang Y, *et al.* What should the government do regarding health policy-making to develop community health care in Shanghai? *Int J Health Plann Manage* 2011; **26(4):** 379–435.

8. Wong SY, Kung K, Griffiths SM, *et al.* Comparison of primary care experiences among adults in general outpatient clinics and private general practice clinics in Hong Kong. *BMC Public Health* 2010; **10:** 397.

9. Goodyear-Smith F, Kassai R. International primary care snapshots: New Zealand and Japan. *Br J Gen Pract* 2015; DOI: 10.3399/bjgp15X684109.

10. Shin DW, Cho J, Yang HK, *et al.* Impact of continuity of care on mortality and health care costs: a nationwide cohort study in Korea. *Ann Fam Med* 2014; **12(6):** 534–541. DOI: 10.1370/afm.1685.

11. Tan CC. National disease management plans for key chronic non-communicable diseases in Singapore. *Ann Acad Med Singapore* 2002; **31(4):** 415–418.

12. Ministry of Health, Singapore. *Primary care survey 2010 report.* https://www.moh.gov.sg/content/moh_web/home/Publications/Reports/2014/primary-care-survey-2010-report.html (accessed 22 Apr 2016).

13. Chen TJ, Chou LF, Hwang SJ. Patterns of ambulatory care utilization in Taiwan. *BMC Health Serv Res* 2006; **6:** 54.

14. Kidd M, ed. *The contribution of family medicine to improving health systems: a guidebook from the World Organization of Family Doctors.* 2nd edn. London, New York: Radcliffe Publishing, 2013.

15. De Maeseneer J, van Weel C, Egilman D, *et al.* Funding for primary health care in developing countries. *BMJ* 2008; **336(7643):** 518–519.

Attribution

Weel C van, Kassai R, Tsoi GWW, Hwang SJ, Cho K, Wong SYS, Chong P-N, Jiang S, Ii M, Goodyear-Smith F. Evolving health policy for primary care in the Asia Pacific region. *British Journal of General Practice* 2016. doi: 10.3399/bjgp16X685513. Reproduced with permission.

CHAPTER 7

East Mediterranean

Chris van Weel, Faisal Alnasir, Taghreed Farahat, Jinan Usta, Mona Osman, Mariam Abdulmalik, Nagwa Nashat, Wadeia Mohamed Alsharief, Salwa Sanousi, Hassan Saleh, Mohammed Tarawneh, Felicity Goodyear-Smith, Amanda Howe and Ryuki Kassai

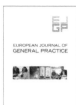

European Journal of General Practice

EUROPEAN JOURNAL OF
GENERAL PRACTICE

ISSN: 1381-4788 (Print) 1751-1402 (Online) Journal homepage: http://www.tandfonline.com/loi/igen20

Primary healthcare policy implementation in the Eastern Mediterranean region: Experiences of six countries

Chris van Weel, Faisal Alnasir, Taghreed Farahat, Jinan Usta, Mona Osman, Mariam Abdulmalik, Nagwa Nashat, Wadeia Mohamed Alsharief, Salwa Sanousi, Hassan Saleh, Mohammed Tarawneh, Felicity Goodyear-Smith, Amanda Howe & Ryuki Kassai

To cite this article: Chris van Weel, Faisal Alnasir, Taghreed Farahat, Jinan Usta, Mona Osman, Mariam Abdulmalik, Nagwa Nashat, Wadeia Mohamed Alsharief, Salwa Sanousi, Hassan Saleh, Mohammed Tarawneh, Felicity Goodyear-Smith, Amanda Howe & Ryuki Kassai (2017): Primary healthcare policy implementation in the Eastern Mediterranean region: Experiences of six countries, European Journal of General Practice, DOI: 10.1080/13814788.2017.1397624

To link to this article: https://doi.org/10.1080/13814788.2017.1397624

Published online: 23 Nov 2017.

Submit your article to this journal ☑

View related articles ☑

View Crossmark data ☑

EUROPEAN JOURNAL OF GENERAL PRACTICE, 2017
https://doi.org/10.1080/13814788.2017.1397624

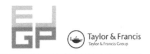

BACKGROUND PAPER

ᵃ OPEN ACCESS   Check for updates

Primary healthcare policy implementation in the Eastern Mediterranean region: Experiences of six countries

Chris van Weel[a,b] , Faisal Alnasir[c] , Taghreed Farahat[d], Jinan Usta[e], Mona Osman[e],
Mariam Abdulmalik[f], Nagwa Nashat[d], Wadeia Mohamed Alsharief[g], Salwa Sanousi[h], Hassan Saleh[i],
Mohammed Tarawneh[j], Felicity Goodyear-Smith[k] , Amanda Howe[l] and Ryuki Kassai[m]

[a]Department of Primary and Community Care, Radboud University Medical Centre, Nijmegen, The Netherlands; [b]Department of
Health Services Research and Policy, Australian National University, Canberra, Australia; [c]Department of Primary Care and Public
Health, Imperial College, London, UK; [d]Department of Family Medicine, Menoufia University, Menoufia, Egypt; [e]Department of Family
Medicine, American University of Beirut, Beirut, Lebanon; [f]Primary Health Care Corporation, Doha, Qatar; [g]Primary Health Care
Services, Dubai Health Authority, Dubai, UAE; [h]Department of Family and Community Medicine, University of Gezira, Gezira, Sudan;
[i]Department of Health System Development, WHO EMR Office, Cairo, Egypt; [j]WONCA East Mediterranean Region, Amman, Jordan;
[k]Department of General Practice and Primary Health Care, University of Auckland, Auckland, New Zealand; [l]Department of Population
Health and Primary Care, University of East Anglia, Norwich, UK; [m]Department of Community and Family Medicine, Fukushima
Medical University, Fukushima, Japan

KEY MESSAGES

- Primary healthcare (PHC) as a policy priority in eastern Mediterranean countries is hampered by policy-makers' lack of understanding the complex nature of PHC.
- Advocacy of PHC should stress its contribution to Universal Health Coverage.
- Professional training in the community setting is a priority to implement PHC.

ABSTRACT

Background: Primary healthcare (PHC) is essential for equitable access and cost-effective health-care. This makes PHC a key factor in the global strategy for universal health coverage (UHC). Implementing PHC requires an understanding of the health system under prevailing circumstances, but for most countries, no data are available.

Objectives: This paper describes and analyses the health systems of Bahrain, Egypt, Lebanon, Qatar, Sudan and the United Arab Emirates, in relation to PHC.

Methods: Data were collected during a workshop at the WONCA East Mediterranean Regional Conference in 2017. Academic family physicians (FP) presented their country, using the WONCA framework of 11 PowerPoint slides with queries of the country demographics, main health challenges, and the position of PHC in the health system.

Results: All six countries have improved the health of their populations, but currently face challenges of non-communicable diseases, aging populations and increasing costs. Main concerns were a lack of trained FPs in community settings, underuse of prevention and of equitable access to care. Countries differed in the extent to which this had resulted in coherent policy.

Conclusion: Priorities were (i) advocacy for community-based PHC to policymakers, including the importance of coordination of healthcare at the community level, and UHC to respond to the needs of populations; (ii) collaboration with universities to include PHC as a core component of every medical curriculum; (iii) collaboration with communities to improve public understanding of PHC; (iv) engagement with the private sector to focus on PHC and UHC.

ARTICLE HISTORY
Received 12 July 2017
Revised 14 September 2017
Accepted 18 October 2017

KEYWORDS
Primary healthcare;
community health
services; family physicians;
healthcare facilities;
healthcare quality; access;
health services

Introduction

Most countries experience significant challenges to their health systems, due to increasing health costs and diminished returns on healthcare investment for aging populations. Where primary healthcare (PHC) is formally structured in the health system, and professionals are educated in the primary care setting, the system realizes better population health at lower

---

CONTACT Chris van Weel Chris.vanWeel@radboudumc.nl Department of Primary and Community Care, Radboud University Medical Centre,
Postbus 9101, 6500 HB Nijmegen, The Netherlands

healthcare costs [1–4]. This has made PHC a global strategy to secure sustainable healthcare [5]. This policy strategy has been reinforced by the pursuit of universal health coverage (UHC) [6], as part of the UN sustainable development goals [7].

Implementing PHC policy asks for the application of general principles under prevailing local conditions [8], and builds PHC from the community level where it operates [9]. An understanding of the existing health system is essential in initiating reforms. This is available for Europe, Australia, New Zealand, and North America [4,8], but for many countries or regions data are scarce [9]. To address this, the World Organization of Family Doctors (WONCA) Working Party on Research took the initiative to document PHC around the world, and stimulate dialogues of how the values of PHC can be addressed within the constraints of different health systems [10]. Earlier studies documented the Asia-Pacific and South Asia regions and in Mexico [11–13]. From these studies, common challenges and priorities were identified to realise PHC and secure UHC— despite differences in culture, demography or history of health systems. This stresses their relevance for other regions, including Europe.

This paper is the first to document and critically appraise the health systems from the Eastern Mediterranean region, with the objective of identifying common strategies for strengthening PHC, and prioritizing regional collaboration, and exploring collaboration with the World Health Organization (WHO) Regional Office for the Eastern Mediterranean (EMR).

Methods

A workshop at the 2017 WONCA East Mediterranean Regional Conference in Abu Dhabi compared the health systems of six WONCA member countries: Bahrain, Egypt, Lebanon, Qatar, Sudan and the United Arab Emirates (UAE) provided the data for this paper. Each selected an academic family physician (FP) to present their country, using the WONCA framework of 11 PowerPoint slides that focused on country demographics, the health system and the position of PHC, the country's leading health challenges, strengths and weaknesses and lessons others could learn from their country [10]. They were free to concentrate on what, in their view, was the most important. All workshop presenters and moderators contributed to the discussion, directed to strategies to strengthen PHC and the contribution regional and international collaboration could make. Presentations (of which presenters provided a summary) and the discussions formed the basis of this article.

Findings: country profiles

Bahrain has a population of 1.4 million served by 9.1 physicians per 10,000 inhabitants, working in the private and government sectors [14,15]. PHC was introduced in the 1950s and strengthened in 1983 through a four-year specialty-training programme for FPs in collaboration with the American University of Beirut, the Irish College of General Practitioners and The Royal College of Surgeons in Ireland. On graduation, each physician has to undergo the Arab Board Examination. This has enhanced the incorporation of the concept of family medicine and its acceptance by the public [16]. Over 24 PHC centres and three clinics have been established in the country geographically, with people registered according to their residential addresses. Health centres differ in the size of the population served, between less than 15,000 to 30,000–35,000. At present around 500 qualified FPs have graduated from the program, but nearly double this number are needed for the growing population. The main problem is the small capacity of the training program of 20 candidates annually.

Egypt has a population of 92.1 million with 28.3 physicians per 10,000 inhabitants [15,17]. PHC was established in the early 1940s based on general practice and maternity and child health services by the mid-1990s. There are approximately 5314 PHC facilities with 14,973 general practitioners and 256 certified FPs. Of these facilities, 61% implemented an FP approach based on formal accreditation [17]. Three types of facilities are in operation: family health units, family health centres, and district hospitals; with a PHC facility within less than 5 km for 95% of the population. This has resulted in nearly 91% children aged 18–29 months fully vaccinated [18]. The government has created a four-year FP fellowship training programme, while various universities did shape a postgraduate five-year training programme and some universities introduced PHC in their undergraduate curriculum. Despite the wide geographic distribution of PHC, there are still only 0.6 PHC centres and units, and less than 0.08 FPs per 10,000 population. The main challenges are the high out-of-pocket expenditure on health, low government spending and poor government vision on family practice, resulting in poor public health services that force most of the poorest to use private healthcare.

Lebanon is has a population of 5.8 million, with 31.9 physicians per 10,000 [15]. The health system is based on a public–private partnership with less than half the population covered by health insurance. The government covers the remaining for secondary and

EUROPEAN JOURNAL OF GENERAL PRACTICE ⓔ 3

tertiary care, while PHC requires out of pocket payment. Private practice dominates, particularly in large cities [19]. There are five FP residency programmes but the number of practicing FPs is limited. There are approximately 950 dispensaries and PHC centres providing affordable healthcare to the poorer segments of the population. The government provides in-kind support to its 200 PHC centres, which are mainly managed by non-governmental organizations or municipalities [20]. Multidisciplinary teams provide comprehensive preventive and curative care (immunizations, child and reproductive care, oral health, provision of essential acute and chronic medications). Strategies taken to strengthen PHC are integrated management of mental health and non-communicable diseases; professional capacity building; accreditation of PHC centres; and introducing a health information system. This has resulted in improved quality and enhanced community engagement [21]. The first steps towards UHC were directed at individuals living below the poverty line. Serious challenges are the limited PHC budget, a further influx of refugees on top of the current one million from Syria [22], and the unstable economic and political situation.

Qatar has a population of 2.4 million, with 77.4 physicians per 10,000 inhabitants [15]. It launched a national health strategy in 2011, with PHC as its basis. This was followed-up by a *Vision* articulating the requirements of a healthy society to meet the country's growth and development. In this, the Prince of Qatar decreed an independent funding and leading role for the PHC Corporation in 2012. The PHC Corporation is now responsible for 23 health centres, all accredited by Accreditation Canada International, in three different regions geographically distributed across the State of Qatar as a public provider. Its focus is on integrating high-quality curative services with promoting healthy living, and on community and patient engagement towards a healthier future. This is based on the family medicine model, through multidisciplinary teams that cover all age groups with a wide range of services (including prevention, management of chronic illness, rehabilitation support, and end of life care) in the community. There are currently 139 certified Qatari FPs, with 12 FPs graduating annually through the FP residency programme—which is insufficient to cover the country's needs. This exemplifies some challenges Qatar is facing but at the same time captures a positive incentive towards PHC.

Sudan with a population of 39.6 million and 2.5 physicians per 10,000 started the PHC approach in 1976 to achieve rural extension for the then urban-based health services [15]. A significant issue is the

shortage of health professionals and their background: there are six times more physicians than nurses, while most of the physicians are specialists (less than one third of generalists). On top of this comes the high turnover: a substantial number of FPs move to Saudi Arabia and the Gulf after graduation. An FP training programme was established in Sudan in 2008. To date, 375 FPs have graduated, of whom 174 still work in the country. In Gezira, there are 120 students enrolled in its FP master programme (with an additional 250 in public health) and 50–60 in Khartoum. Its programme pursues a family health approach led by three categories of PHC providers: FPs, medical assistants, and community health workers who operate basic health units and deliver essential PHC services. The health centre headed by FPs forms the first referral point for lower-level facilities. The community participates in the planning and performance of PHC. Currently, 109 FPs work in 84 health centres.

The UAE has an estimated population of 9.6 million of which Emirati nationals represent 19% [15]. Population growth and aging, together with an increase of medical tourism stretch the available facilities [23]. There are 19.3 physicians and 40.9 nurses and midwives per 10,000 inhabitants and well over 104 public and private hospitals and 1075 public and private outpatient clinics [15,24]. This includes 150 public centres and clinics, that provide PHC and in which 1004 physicians (363 residency trained FPs) practice with a further 40 PHC centres planned [25]. This has resulted in substantial progress in population health, in particular maternity and infant health, with all births attended by skilled health professionals. The FP residency training established in Dubai in 1993 is now extended to Al Ain, Abu-Dhabi, and Sharjah and the northern Emirates with four-year programmes recognized by the Arab Board of Medical Specialization. Collaboration with the UK Royal College of General Practitioners has improved the quality of these programmes. The annual output of the FP residency training programmes of 16 is insufficient to meet the demands of the UAE now and in the short-term, while the introduction of universal health insurance will further increase this demand.

Discussion

Each country presented a unique situation, but all had PHC on their health agenda. From it, four themes emerged: (i) the gap between PHC facilities currently realized and what is required to serve their populations; (ii) problems amongst policymakers in understanding the complex nature of PHC and the importance of comprehensive policy to realize it;

(iii) the importance of investing in the training of (future) professionals in the primary healthcare setting; and (iv) the importance of involving the private, next to the public sector in health reforms.

All six countries have made progress in the health of their populations but there were general concerns of an underuse of prevention and of equitable access to care. Countries differed in the realization of a coherent policy to address these issues. Bahrain and Sudan have developed a structure of community based PHC as the entry point of the health system, with a leading role for FPs, and Qatar has recently launched plans to strengthen community engagement in improving health outcomes. In Lebanon, the introduction of UHC is connected to the provision of community health services and directed at the poorest population. Other countries are aware of the need to introduce PHC in their health systems, but without a targeted policy to bring this about. This was exemplified in Egypt, with its long tradition of PHC that has improved maternity and child health [17]. Yet, as had also been seen in other regions, the successful implementation of *limited PHC* (i.e. restricted to programs focussing on only a few health problems) has not evolved in a structure that integrates the broad field of prevention, treatment and support of all health problems in all individuals [12].

Implications: integrated health policy

To achieve this integrated approach, a comprehensive health policy is required to regulate the health system, define the role and function of PHC, and make sure that professionals have the competence to fulfil this role. Of particular importance is here to include the private sector [25], as most healthcare (including that for the poorest segment of the population) is provided privately [26]. Public–private partnerships are common in the region, but not in health policy. Regulation and standardization of the private sector is required to stimulate collaboration and promotion of health, to address the needs of the populations. Related to this, PHC has to have the function to coordinate and horizontally integrate the provision of healthcare. Health policy should counter that every specialist can claim 'primary health care' and practice in the community.

Implications: professional capacity building

For PHC to be able to lead the health system, training of professionals—including FPs—in the PHC setting is a mandatory precondition. Specialty training for FPs is provided by medical schools in the countries, but has a low priority, resulting in a shortage of FPs [27]. The

strong focus on secondary and hospital-based care, with its high status amongst patients and public has been encountered in other regions as well [28]. Those who have completed specialty training experience their competences undervalued, which further stimulates a 'brain drain' to other countries and regions.

Another measure is to combine programmes for practitioners already working in the system to improve their skills with specialty training of residents, as recommended by the WHO EMRO [27].

Implications: understanding PHC

For consistent policy, it is essential to understand the complex nature of PHC and of how it contributes to health systems. Unfortunately, policymakers consider PHC an ill-understood 'black box' [29], and that is where WHO EMRO has focussed its advocacy and where academic and professional PHC organizations can make a valuable contribution [27].

Implications: towards regional collaboration

The shared challenges on the road to PHC implementation present a strong case for regional collaboration in which PHC leadership connects with policymakers and other stakeholders [25,30]. In this, a partnership with the powerful WHO EMRO office would offer an excellent opportunity for a regional action plan to realize UHC through PHC [26,27].

The priorities in PHC that emerged from this analysis concur with priorities in other regions—including Europe. Particularly relevant from a European perspective is how to align the private and public sectors in PHC development and how to secure a policy towards UHC that comprehensively addresses the health system regulations, professionals' roles, and specialty training.

Conclusion and key messages

Despite their differences in their socio-economic situation and track record of their health systems, the six countries face the same challenges in securing robust PHC and UHC. In conclusion, four priorities of joint action were identified:

- Advocacy for community-based PHC and UHC to policymakers, including the central role of PHC in coordinating healthcare at the community level. The experiences in Bahrain and Sudan can serve as models of success;
- Collaboration with university leaders and deans of medical schools to include PHC as a core

component of every medical curriculum, followed by specialty training in PHC settings for those choosing a career as FP;

- Collaboration with patients and community leaders to inform the public about the role and function of PHC to improve its understanding. Collecting and displaying stories and experiences of patients can be of great value in this [13].
- As the private sector is a main outpatient health services provider, engaging the private health sector is inevitable to realize UHC.

Disclosure statement

The authors report no conflicts of interest. The authors alone are responsible for the content and writing of this article.

ORCID

Chris van Weel http://orcid.org/0000-0003-3653-4701
Faisal Alnasir http://orcid.org/0000-0002-5840-5081
Felicity Goodyear-Smith http://orcid.org/0000-0002-6657-9401

References

[1] Starfield B. Is primary care essential? Lancet. 1994;344: 1129–1133.

[2] Starfield B, Shi L, Macinko J. Contribution of primary care to health systems and health. Milbank Q. 2005;83:457–502.

[3] Hansen J, Groenewegen PP, Boerma GW, et al. Living in a country with a strong primary care system is beneficial to people with chronic conditions. Health Aff (Millwood). 2015;34:1531–1537.

[4] Kringos D, The strength of primary care in Europe [thesis]. Utrecht, University of Utrecht, 2012 [Internet]; [cited 2017 Feb 28]. Available from: http://www.nivel.nl/sites/default/files/bestanden/Proefschrift-Dionne-Kringos-The-strength-of-primary-care.pdf

[5] World Health Organization. The World Health Report 2008: primary health care, now more than ever. Geneva: WHO; 2008 [Internet]; [cited 2017 Feb 28]. Available from: http://www.who.int/whr/2008/en/

[6] United Nations. Sustainable Development Goals. 2017. [Internet]; [cited 2017 Apr 19]. Available from: http://www.un.org/sustainabledevelopment/sustainable-development-goals/

[7] WHO. Universal Health Coverage. 2017. [Internet]; [cited 2017 Feb 13]. Available from: http://www.who.int/universal_health_coverage/en/

[8] Journal of the American Board of Family Medicine. 2012;25(Suppl 1). [Internet]; [cited 2017 Mar 4] Available from: http://www.jabfm.org/content/25/Suppl_1.toc

[9] van Weel C, Turnbull D, Whitehead E, et al. International collaboration in innovating health systems. Ann Fam Med. 2015;13:86–87.

[10] WONCA research working party multi-national plenary panel project. 2017. [Internet]; [cited 2017 March 04]. Available from: http://www.globalfamilydoctor.com/groups/WorkingParties/Research/plenarypanelprojec-tresourcedocuments.aspx

[11] van Weel C, Kassai R, Tsoi GWW, et al. Evolving health policy for primary care in the Asia Pacific region. Br J Gen Pract. 2016;66:e451–e453.

[12] van Weel C, Kassai R, Qidwai W, et al. Primary health-care policy implementation in South Asia. BMJ Glob Health. 2016;1:e000057.

[13] van Weel C, Turnbull D, Ramirez J, et al. Supporting health reforms in Mexico: experiences and suggestions from an international primary health care conference. Ann Fam Med. 2016;14:280–281.

[14] Alnasir F. Ageing and pattern of population changes in the developing countries. MEJAA. 2015;12:26–32.

[15] WHO EMRO. Country health profiles. 2017. [Internet]; [cited 2017 Sep 6]. Available from: http://www.emro.who.int/entity/statistics/statistics.html

[16] Alnasir F. Family medicine in the Arab world? Is it a luxury? J Bahrain Med Soc. 2009;21:191–192.

[17] Government of Egypt. CAPMAS statistical yearbook (after MOHP). 2016. [Internet]; [cited 2017 Mar 23]. Available from: http://www.capmas.gov.eg/Pages/StaticPages.aspx?page_id=5034

[18] El-Zanaty F, et al. Egypt Demographic and Health Survey 2014. Cairo and Maryland: Ministry of Health and Population, the DHS Program, ICF International, 2014. [Internet]; Available from: http://dhsprogram.com/pubs/pdf/PR54/PR54.pdf

[19] World Health Organization. Country cooperation strategy for WHO and Lebanon 2010–2015. 2017. [Internet]; [cited 2017 Mar 23]. Available from: http://www.who.int/country-cooperation/publications/en/

[20] Ammar W, Kdouh O, Hammoud R, et al. Health system reliance: Lebanon and the Syrian refugee crisis. J Glob Health. 2016;6:020704.

[21] El-Jardali F, Hemadeh R, Jaafar M, et al. The impact of accreditation of primary health care centres: successes, challenges and policy implications as perceived by primary health care providers and directors in Lebanon. BMC Health Serv Res. 2014;14:86.

[22] United Nations High Commissioner on Refugees. Syria Regional Refugee Response. Inter-agency information sharing portal. Syria: UNHCR 2017. [Internet]; [cited 2017 Mar 23]. Available from: http://data.unhcr.org/syrianrefugees/country.php?id=122

[23] Gulf News. March 30, 2017. Dubai prepares for influx of 1.3 m medical tourists by 2021. 2017. [Internet]; [cited 2017 Mar 30]. Available from: http://gulfnews.com/news/uae/health/dubai-prepares-for-influx-of-1-3m-medical-tourists-by-2021-1.1818558

[24] The U.S.–U.A.E. Business Council. The U.A.E. healthcare sector: an update. September 2016. [Internet]; [cited 2017 Mar 30]. Available from: http://usuaebusiness.org/wp-content/uploads/2016/09/Healthcare-Report-Final.pdf

[25] UAE Interact. 2017. [Internet]; [cited 2017 Mar 30]. Available from: http://www.uaeinteract.com/society/health.asp

[26] World Health Organization. Regional Office for the Eastern Mediterranean. Analysis of the private health sector in countries of the Eastern Mediterranean. 2014. [Internet]; [cited 2014 Apr 03]. Available from: http://applications.emro.who.int/dsaf/EMROPUB_2014_EN_1790.pdf?ua=1

[27] Scaling up family practice: progressing towards universal health coverage, EM/RC63/Tech.Disc.1. 2016. [Internet]; [cited 2017 Sept 04]. Available from: http://www.emro.who.int/about-who/rc63/documentation.html

[28] van Weel C, Kassai R. Expanding primary care in South and East Asia. BMJ. 2017;356:j634.

[29] Primary Health Care Performance Initiative. 2017 Measuring PHC. [Internet]; [cited 2017 Mar 8]. Available from: http://phcperformanceinitiative.org/about-us/measuring-phc

[30] Rawaf S, Qidwai W, Khoja TAM, et al. New leadership model for family physicians in the Eastern Mediterranean region: a pilot study across selected countries. J Fam Med. 2017;4:1107.

Attribution

Chris van W, Faisal A, Taghreed F, Jinan U, Mona O, Mariam A, Nagwa N, Wadeia M.A, Salwa S, Hassan S, Mohammed T, Felicity G-S, Amanda H, Ryuki K. Primary health care policy implementation in the East Mediterranean region – Experiences of six countries. *European Journal of General Practice* 2017;23. doi: 10.1080/13814788.2017.1397624. Reproduced with permission.

CHAPTER 8

Europe

Willemijn L.A. Schäfer, Wienke G.W. Boerma, Anna M. Murante, Herman J.M. Sixma, François G. Schellevis and Peter P. Groenewegen

Assessing the potential for improvement of primary care in 34 countries: a cross-sectional survey

Willemijn LA Schäfer,[a] Wienke GW Boerma,[a] Anna M Murante,[b] Herman JM Sixma,[a] François G Schellevis[a] & Peter P Groenewegen[a]

Objective To investigate patients' perceptions of improvement potential in primary care in 34 countries.

Methods We did a cross-sectional survey of 69 201 patients who had just visited general practitioners at primary-care facilities. Patients rated five features of person-focused primary care – accessibility/availability, continuity, comprehensiveness, patient involvement and doctor–patient communication. One tenth of the patients ranked the importance of each feature on a scale of one to four, and nine tenths of patients scored their experiences of care received. We calculated the potential for improvement by multiplying the proportion of negative patient experiences with the mean importance score in each country. Scores were divided into low, medium and high improvement potential. Pair-wise correlations were made between improvement scores and three dimensions of the structure of primary care – governance, economic conditions and workforce development.

Findings In 26 countries, one or more features of primary care had medium or high improvement potentials. Comprehensiveness of care had medium to high improvement potential in 23 of 34 countries. In all countries, doctor–patient communication had low improvement potential. An overall stronger structure of primary care was correlated with a lower potential for improvement of continuity and comprehensiveness of care. In countries with stronger primary care governance patients perceived less potential to improve the continuity of care. Countries with better economic conditions for primary care had less potential for improvement of all features of person-focused care.

Conclusion In countries with a stronger primary care structure, patients perceived that primary care had less potential for improvement.

Abstracts in عربي, 中文, Français, Русский and Español at the end of each article.

Introduction

Due to the increased prevalence of comorbid conditions, people often have more than one disease that needs to be managed consistently over time.[1,2] Health-care providers can do this through a person-focused approach, which entails goal-oriented, rather than disease-oriented care. The goal is to manage people's illnesses through the course of their life.[1,2] Therefore, person-focused care should be continuous, accessible and comprehensive. It should also be coordinated when patients have more than one provider.[3]

Patients' assessment of health care can be divided into what patients find important and what they have experienced.[3–5] Importance refers to what people see as desired features of health care – i.e. patients' instrumental values.[6] The combination of instrumental values and patients' experiences constitute quality judgments, which provides insight on the extent to which health-care providers meet these values. Both instrumental values and experiences of primary care patients vary between countries.[6–8] These judgements can be transformed into a measure of improvement potential. When an aspect of care is experienced as poorly performed, but not considered important, this can be seen as less of a quality problem than if patients consider the aspect important.[9] More important aspects of care thus have higher improvement potential.

The structure of primary care can relate to person-focused care in various ways. In stronger primary care structures the providers are more likely to be involved in a wide range of health problems at different stages of the patients' lives. This is expected to increase continuity of care and providers'

responsiveness to the patients' values regarding continuity, comprehensiveness and communication. Patients will use services more readily if they know a broad spectrum of care is offered.[10] A stronger primary care structure is associated with more accessible primary care,[11] which is one of the core features of person-focused care. Therefore, we expect that in countries with a stronger primary care structure, the patient-perceived improvement potential of person-focused primary care is lower.

The primary care structure comprises governance, economic conditions such as the mode of financing of providers and expenditures on primary care, and workforce development – the profile and the education of the primary-care providers.[12,13]

We wished to quantify the extent to which the structure of primary care at the national level in 34 countries is related to patient-perceived improvement potential for features of person-focused care. To study this relationship, the empirical relations between the providers – general practitioners – and patients need to be considered (Fig. 1). The primary care structure influences the behaviour of the practitioners, which will influence patients' experiences. Patients' characteristics – e.g. age and income – influence patients' individual experiences and values. We focus on the system level to study characteristics that are amenable to policy interventions.

Methods

We derived aggregated data on patient-perceived improvement potential in 34 countries from the QUALICOPC study (Quality and Costs of Primary Care in Europe). In this study, patients

a NIVEL, Netherlands Institute for Health Services Research, PO Box 1568, 3500 BN Utrecht, Netherlands.
b Scuola Superiore Sant'Anna, Istituto di Management, Pisa, Italy.
Correspondence to Willemijn LA Schäfer (email: w.schafer@nivel.nl).

(Submitted: 22 April 2014 – Revised version received: 10 December 2014 – Accepted: 18 December 2014 – Published online: 28 January 2015)

Fig. 1. **Features that influence the extent to which primary care is person-focused**

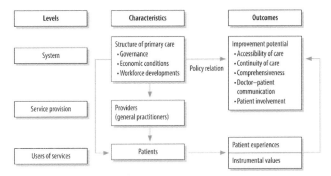

Note: Instrumental value is what the patient finds important.

in 31 European countries (Austria, Belgium, Bulgaria, Cyprus, Czech Republic, Denmark, Estonia, Finland, Germany, Greece, Hungary, Iceland, Ireland, Italy, Latvia, Lithuania, Luxembourg, Malta, the Netherlands, Norway, Poland, Portugal, Romania, Slovakia, Slovenia, Spain, Sweden, Switzerland, the former Yugoslav Republic of Macedonia, Turkey, the United Kingdom of Great Britain and Northern Ireland) responded to surveys. Three non-European countries (Australia, Canada, New Zealand) were also included. In each country, patients of general practitioners filled in the questionnaires (target: $n = 2200$ per country; Cyprus, Iceland and Luxembourg $n = 800$). In Belgium, Canada, Spain and Turkey, larger samples were taken to enable comparisons between regions (Table 1). We aimed to get a nationally representative sample of general practitioners. If national registers of practitioners were available, we used random sampling to select practitioners. In countries with only regional registers, random samples were drawn from regions that represented the national setting. If no registers existed, but only lists of facilities in a country, a random selection from such lists was made. The patients of only one practitioner per practice or health centre were eligible to participate. Details of the study protocol have been published elsewhere.[14,15]

In nearly all countries (30), trained fieldworkers were sent to the participating practices to collect patient data using paper questionnaires. In Canada, Denmark, New Zealand, the United Kingdom and parts of Norway

and Sweden, the practice staff were instructed to distribute and collect the questionnaires. The fieldworkers and practice staff were instructed to invite consecutive patients, who had had a face-to-face consultation with the practitioner and who were 18 years or older, to complete the questionnaire until 10 questionnaires per practice were collected. Of these 10 questionnaires, nine assessed the experiences in the consultation which had just occurred and one questionnaire included questions about the patient's primary care values. The proportions of the questionnaires were based on the findings that, within a country, patients' experiences varied widely but there was little variation in what the patients found important.[7] In the patient experience questionnaire, patients were asked to indicate whether they agreed with a statement by selecting "Yes" or "No" answers. For example, the proportion of negative experiences for the statement "during the consultation the doctor had my medical records at hand" would be the proportion stating that the doctor did not have the medical records at hand. In the patient values' questionnaire – which contained the same questions as the patient experience questionnaire – patients could indicate the importance of a statement, e.g. the importance of the doctor having medical records at hand, by selecting "not important", "somewhat important", "important" or "very important". The answers were scored, ranging from 1 (not important) to 4 (very important). Missing answers were excluded from the calculations.

Ethical approval was acquired in accordance with the legal requirements in each country. The surveys were carried out anonymously. Data collection took place between October 2011 and December 2013. The patient experience questionnaire was filled in by 61 931 patients and the patient values' questionnaire by 7270 patients. Appendices A and B contain the questionnaires (available at: http://www.nivel.nl/pdf/Appendices-Assesing-the-potential-for-improvement-of-PC-in-34-countries-WHO-Bulletin-2015.pdf).

Operationalization of concepts

Dependent variables

As an outcome indicator for health care, we used the patient-perceived improvement potential, which is based on the consumer quality (CQ) index, a validated and standardized measurement instrument.[16] Person-focused primary care was measured using 16 items, such as whether the practitioner displayed knowledge about the patient's personal living circumstances. The items were derived from the CQ index for general practice and tested in the QUALICOPC pilot study.[15,17] Improvement potential was expressed in improvement scores, which are calculated by multiplying the proportion of negative experiences for each question – the answers which indicate lower quality – with the value scores of the corresponding statement per country. The value score was calculated by taking the mean value for each country on a scale from one to four. A higher improvement score indicates a higher need for improvement.

The improvement potential of each country was measured for the following main features: accessibility/availability (five questions), continuity (three questions), comprehensiveness (two questions), patient involvement (one question) and doctor–patient communication (five questions). For each feature, a mean patient-perceived improvement score was calculated. Based on the range of scores found (0.11–1.95) the level of improvement potential is considered relatively low (0.11–0.72), medium (0.73–1.34) or high (1.35–1.95).

Independent variables

For 30 countries (Australia, Canada, New Zealand and the former Yugoslav Republic of Macedonia were

Willemijn LA Schäfer et al.

Table 1. **Overview of the survey investigating the potential for improvement of primary care in 34 countries, 2011–2013**

Country	No. of general practitioners facilities[a]	No. of patient experience questionnaires completed	No. of patient values' questionnaires completed	Relative strength of primary care structure[b]
Australia	133	1190	138	Strong
Austria	180	1596	188	Medium
Belgium	411	3677	407	Medium
Bulgaria	221	1991	222	Weak
Canada	553	5009	806	Strong
Cyprus	71	624	71	Weak
Czech Republic	220	1980	220	Weak
Denmark	212	1878	209	Strong
Estonia	128	1121	126	Medium
Finland	139	1196	129	Medium
Germany	237	2117	234	Medium
Greece	221	1964	219	Weak
Hungary	221	1934	215	Weak
Iceland	90	761	82	Weak
Ireland	191	1694	186	Medium
Italy	219	1959	220	Strong
Latvia	218	1951	212	Medium
Lithuania	225	2011	224	Medium
Luxembourg	80	713	79	Weak
Malta	70	626	68	Weak
Netherlands	228	2012	222	Strong
New Zealand	131	1150	197	Strong
Norway	203	1529	175	Medium
Poland	220	1975	219	Weak
Portugal	212	1920	215	Strong
Romania	220	1975	220	Strong
Slovakia	220	1918	220	Weak
Slovenia	219	1963	216	Strong
Spain	433	3731	431	Strong
Sweden	88	773	112	Medium
Switzerland	200	1791	198	Weak
The former Yugoslav Republic of Macedonia	143	1283	143	Medium
Turkey	290	2623	292	Medium
United Kingdom[c]	160	1296	155	Strong

[a] Patients of one general practitioner per facility were surveyed.
[b] Based on Kringos et al. 2013.
[c] Only patients in England were surveyed.

excluded), we collected data from the Primary Health Care Activity Monitor (PHAMEU) study on a set of indicators for the dimensions of governance, economic conditions and workforce development of the primary care structure.[18] Examples of such indicators are the availability of evidence-based guidelines for general practitioners (governance) and the percentage of medical universities with a postgraduate programme in family medicine (workforce development).[18] The PHAMEU database provides scores indicating the strength of each indicator, ranging from 1 (weak) to 3 (strong) and overall scale scores for each dimension, calculated using a two-level hierarchical latent regression model, and an overall structure score combining the three dimensions.[11] Additionally, we collected data for Australia, Canada, New Zealand and the former Yugoslav Republic of Macedonia using the same methods as for the PHAMEU study. Table 1 lists the relative strength of each countries' primary care structure, Appendix C contains the indicators and Appendix D contains scale scores per dimension.

Statistical analyses

One-tailed pairwise correlations were used to measure the associations between the independent and dependent variables, because the hypothesis has one direction, namely that a stronger primary care structure is associated with more person-focused care. $P < 0.05$ was considered statistically significant.

Sensitivity analyses were done using an alternative method of analysis for the improvement scores. Multilevel analyses were used to calculate country-level scores of the experience and values items, using the country level residuals of the items. The scores were adjusted for several variables at the practitioner and patient level (e.g. age and gender of the general practitioners and patients). When comparing the raw improvement scores and the ones calculated on the basis of multilevel residuals no significant differences were found. Correlation coefficients between the raw improvement scores as used in this paper and the adjusted improvement scores were above 0.91.

In the PHAMEU conceptual model and corresponding database, gatekeeping (practitioners determining the necessity for referral of patients to other levels of the health system) is considered to be part of the process of primary care. However, in previous studies, gatekeeping has been used as a potential determinant of primary care performance. Therefore, additional sensitivity analysis was performed on the association between the improvement potential and gatekeeping. The results of this analysis are presented in Appendix E. Analyses were carried out using Stata version 13.0 (StataCorp. LP, College Station, United States of America) and MLWin version 2.25 (University of Bristol, Bristol, United Kingdom).

Results

Improvement potential

In total, 69 201 patients completed the questionnaire and the average response rate was 74.1% (range: 54.5%–87.6%). A detailed overview of the patients' experience scores, values' scores and patient-perceived improvement scores per country are provided in Appendices F–H. The background characteristics of the patients can be found in Appendix I.

For accessibility of care, five countries – Cyprus, Portugal, Slovakia, Spain and Turkey – showed a medium level of improvement potential. The remaining countries showed a low improvement potential. While most of the countries were found to have a low improvement potential regarding the continuity of care, Greece, Malta and Turkey show a medium level and Cyprus a high level. Comprehensiveness of care showed a medium level of patient-perceived improvement potential in 20 countries and a relatively high level in Cyprus, Malta and Sweden. Patients' involvement in decision-making about their treatment had a medium level of improvement potential in nine countries and a high level in Cyprus. In all countries, values were relatively low for doctor–patient communication, indicating that the primary-care providers meet their patients' expectations in this domain (Table 2).

The relatively high levels of patient-perceived improvement potential in Cyprus – three features with high potential and one feature with medium – indicate weak performance of primary care. In Turkey, three areas showed a medium level of patient-perceived improvement potential. Countries showing relatively low improvement potential in all features were Australia, Belgium, Canada, Ireland, Latvia, Luxembourg, New Zealand and Switzerland, indicating that primary care in these countries is perceived as person-focused.

Table 2. **Mean patient-perceived improvement scores for primary care in 34 countries, 2011–2013**

Country	Improvement score[a]				
	Accessibility	Continuity	Comprehensiveness	Involvement	Communication
Australia	0.38	0.14	0.42	0.17	0.16
Austria	0.41	0.38	0.97	0.65	0.20
Belgium	0.34	0.26	0.57	0.26	0.22
Bulgaria	0.66	0.56	1.34	1.17	0.34
Canada	0.38	0.11	0.52	0.18	0.12
Cyprus	1.25	1.40	1.95	1.47	0.38
Czech Republic	0.44	0.26	1.00	0.79	0.18
Denmark	0.26	0.18	0.82	0.56	0.23
Estonia	0.40	0.22	0.87	0.80	0.22
Finland	0.46	0.36	0.81	0.55	0.21
Germany	0.33	0.27	0.81	0.50	0.20
Greece	0.72	1.08	0.70	0.77	0.24
Hungary	0.49	0.49	1.05	0.48	0.30
Iceland	0.53	0.24	1.14	0.46	0.24
Ireland	0.45	0.26	0.72	0.66	0.37
Italy	0.51	0.31	0.91	0.76	0.42
Latvia	0.51	0.26	0.67	0.70	0.40
Lithuania	0.52	0.38	0.62	0.84	0.24
Luxembourg	0.39	0.31	0.62	0.57	0.23
Malta	0.60	1.17	1.36	0.65	0.33
Netherlands	0.30	0.25	0.91	0.47	0.28
New Zealand	0.22	0.11	0.52	0.18	0.12
Norway	0.52	0.31	0.93	0.52	0.21
Poland	0.55	0.56	1.02	0.90	0.23
Portugal	0.73	0.19	0.50	0.73	0.27
Romania	0.55	0.30	1.04	0.65	0.29
Slovakia	0.74	0.53	1.12	0.63	0.28
Slovenia	0.53	0.32	1.16	0.78	0.23
Spain	0.90	0.29	1.16	0.57	0.36
Sweden	0.54	0.62	1.38	0.60	0.27
Switzerland	0.27	0.18	0.60	0.27	0.16
The former Yugoslav Republic of Macedonia	0.38	0.23	0.92	0.61	0.14
Turkey	0.77	0.84	1.06	0.38	0.36
United Kingdom[b]	0.42	0.30	0.77	0.47	0.21

[a] The improvement score was calculated by multiplying the proportion of negative patient experiences with the mean importance score.
[b] Only patients in England were surveyed.
Note: Scores between 0.11–0.72 were considered as a low level of patient-perceived improvement potential. Scores between 0.73–1.34 were considered as a medium level of patient-perceived improvement potential. Scores between 1.35–1.95 were considered as a high level of patient-perceived improvement potential.

Primary care structure

The patient-perceived improvement potential for continuity and comprehensiveness of care had a significant negative association with the overall structure of primary care. If a country has a stronger primary care structure, primary care is more person-focused for these features. For the separate structural dimensions, patients' perceived care to be more continuous in countries with stronger primary care governance. Stronger economic conditions in primary care were found to be associated with all features of person-focused care. Although workforce development correlated negatively with all features, none of the values were significantly correlated (Table 3).

In eight countries where patient-perceived improvement potential is relatively low, the overall strength of the primary care structure varies. The relative strength is strong in Australia, Canada and New Zealand, medium in Belgium, Ireland and Latvia and weak in Luxembourg and Switzerland. The strongest associations between strength and improvement potential were found for economic conditions for primary care. These conditions are relatively strong in Australia, Belgium and New Zealand and medium in Latvia and Switzerland.

Discussion

This study evaluates the extent to which primary care in 34 countries is person-focused by asking patients of general practitioners about what they find important and their actual experiences. The combination of these aspects provides us with insight on what patients perceive as priority improvement areas. In most countries primary care shows one or more features with a medium or high level of patient-perceived improvement potential. Accessibility and continuity of care show relatively low improvement potential, while in many countries comprehensiveness is indicated as a priority area. In this study, comprehensiveness of care indicates whether general practitioners ask their patients about additional problems and whether there is opportunity to discuss psychosocial problems. Our results confirm previous studies showing that practitioners perform well on general aspects of communication.[19-21] One ex-

Table 3. **Correlations between the strength of primary care structure and patient perceived improvement scores in 34 countries, 2011–2013**

Feature	Primary care structure			
	Overall	Governance	Economic conditions	Workforce development
Accessibility	−0.2562	−0.1136	−0.3187*	−0.2244
Continuity	−0.3962*	−0.3320*	−0.3833*	−0.2263
Comprehensiveness	−0.3230*	−0.1739	−0.3663*	−0.269
Involvement	−0.2833	−0.0484	−0.5768*	−0.2772
Communication	−0.1202	−0.0475	−0.3720*	−0.0513

*$P < 0.05$ (one-tailed).

planation for this result could be the ongoing relationship between practitioners and their patients. Larger variations have been found between countries on the relevance of communication and practitioners' performance for specific issues.[22] Eight countries showed low improvement potential in all features, indicating positive patient experiences. Previous studies in Australia and New Zealand have also found positive patient experiences.[23,24] Another study comparing 10 European countries, found positive patient assessments in Belgium, Germany and Switzerland and less positive assessments in the United Kingdom and the Scandinavian countries.[21] This is largely in line with our findings.

We could largely confirm the hypothesis that a stronger primary care structure is associated with more person-focused care. Stronger structures were associated with more continuous and comprehensive care. Continuity is an important aspect of person-focused care. Stronger governance is also associated with more continuity. In countries with stronger economic conditions for primary care we found less improvement potential in all areas.

The sensitivity analysis for the association between gatekeeping and patient-perceived improvement potential showed that gatekeeping was associated only with lower perceived improvement potential for continuity of care.

Strengths of this study were the inclusion of data from many countries and that patients were asked about their actual experiences immediately after the consultation with their practitioners. There were also limitations. First, there are countries where other providers offer primary care besides general practitioners. These providers were not included in this study. Second, only the actual visitors to general practices were

surveyed. This means that we do not have information about the people who do not have access to such practices. In all countries, improvement potential for accessibility of care might be higher than measured in this study. For example, a report based on the Canadian QUALICOPC data found that patient-reported access in this study is more positive compared to other previous studies.[25-28] Third, in Greece, most participating general practitioners worked in health centres, while there are also many practitioners in Greece working outside health centres. Comparing different countries should be done cautiously, since the extent to which general practitioners are involved in primary care and the types of illnesses they treat differs between countries.

When measuring instrumental values and experiences of patients, people may judge importance by what they have already experienced in health care.[5] For example, when practitioners in a country perform poorly on a certain aspect, patients might have lower expectations and will find this aspect less important. Experiences and values of patients have been found to be correlated,[5] perhaps because patients seek health-care providers who deliver care according to their values.

The World Health Organization advocates for primary care that puts people first. A stronger primary care structure is necessary to make progress towards this goal.[16] ∎

Acknowledgements

We thank partners in the QUALICOPC project; J De Maeseneer, E De Ryck, L Hanssens, A Van Pottelberge, S Willems (Belgium); S Greß, S Heinemann (Germany); G Capitani, S De Rosis, AM Murante, S Nuti, C Seghieri, M Vainieri (Italy); D Kringos (the

Netherlands); M Van den Berg, T Van Loenen (the Netherlands); D Rotar Pavlič, I Švab (Slovenia).

We thank the coordinators of the data collection in each country: L Jorm, I McRae (Australia); K Hoffmann, M Maier (Austria); P Salchev (Bulgaria); W Wodchis, W Hogg (Canada); G Samoutis (Cyprus); B Seifert, N Šrámková (Czech Republic); J Reinholdt Jensen, P Vedsted (Denmark); M Lember, K Põlluste (Estonia); E Kosunen (Finland); C Lionis (Greece); I Rurik (Hungary); J Heimisdóttir, O Thorgeirsson (Iceland); C Collins (Ireland); G Ticmane (Latvia);

S Macinskas (Lithuania); M Aubart, J Leners, R Stein (Luxembourg); G Bezzina, P Sciortino (Malta); T Ashton, R McNeill (New Zealand); T Bjerve Eide, H Melbye (Norway); M Oleszczyk, A Windak (Poland); L Pisco (Portugal), D Farcasanu (Romania); E Jurgova (Slovakia); T Dedeu (Spain); C Björkelund, T Faresjö (Sweden); T Bisschoff, N Senn (Switzerland); K Stavric (The former Yugoslav Republic of Macedonia); M Akman (Turkey); C Sirdifield, N Siriwardena (United Kingdom).

FGS is also affiliated with the department of General Practice and

Elderly Care Medicine/EMGO Institute for Health and Care Research, VU University Medical Centre, Amsterdam, the Netherlands. PPG is also affiliated with the department of Sociology and the department of Human Geography, Utrecht University, Utrecht, the Netherlands.

Funding: This article is based on the QUALICOPC project, co- funded by the European Commission under the Seventh Framework Programme (FP7/2007-2013) under grant agreement 242141.

Competing interests: None declared.

ملخص

تقييم احتمالات تحسين الرعاية الأولية في 34 بلداً: مسح متعدد القطاعات

الغرض تحري تصورات المرضى حول احتمالات التحسين في مجال الرعاية الأولية في 34 بلداً.

الطريقة أجرينا مسحاً متعدد القطاعات على 69201 مريضاً قاموا للتو بزيارة المارسين العموميين في مرافق الرعاية الأولية. وقام المرضى بتقييم خمس سمات للرعاية الأولية الشخصية – التوافر/ الإتاحة والاستمرارية والشمولية وإشراك المرضى والتواصل بين الأطباء والمرضى. وقام عُشر المرضى بترتيب أهمية كل سمة من السمات باستخدام مقياس من واحد إلى أربعة وسجل تسعة أعشار المرضى خبراتهم بشأن تلقي الرعاية. وقمنا بحساب احتمالات التحسين بضرب نسبة الخبرات السلبية للمرضى بمتوسط درجة الأهمية في كل بلد. وتم تقسيم الدرجات إلى احتمالات تحسين منخفضة ومتوسطة ومرتفعة. وتم إيجاد الارتباطات الثنائية بين درجات التحسين والأبعاد الثلاثة لهيكل الرعاية الأولية وهي – تصريف الشؤون والظروف الاقتصادية وتنمية القوى العاملة.

النتائج حظيت واحدة أو أكثر من سمات الرعاية الأولية في 26 بلداً باحتمالات تحسين متوسطة أو مرتفعة. وحظيت شمولية الرعاية باحتمالات تحسين من متوسطة إلى مرتفعة في 23 بلدا من أصل 34 بلداً. وفي جميع البلدان، حظي التواصل بين الأطباء والمرضى باحتمالات تحسين منخفضة. وارتبط ازدياد هيكل الرعاية الأولية الأقوى بشكل عام بانخفاض احتمالات التحسين في الاستمرارية وشمولية الرعاية. وكان تصور المرضى في البلدان التي تتميز بتصريف شؤون أقوى فيما يتعلق بالرعاية الأولية هو انخفاض احتمالات التحسين في استمرارية الرعاية. وانخفضت احتمالات التحسين في جميع سمات الرعاية الشخصية لدى البلدان ذات الظروف الاقتصادية الأفضل للرعاية الأولية.

الاستنتاج في البلدان ذات هيكل الرعاية الأولية الأقوى، تتسم الرعاية الأولية باحتمالات تحسين أقل وفق تصورات المرضى.

摘要

评估 34 个国家初级保健进行改善的可能性：横断面调查

目的 调查 34 个国家病人对初级保健改善可能性的看法。

方法 我们对最近前往初级保健设施的全科医生就医的 69201 名患者进行横断面调查。病人以个人为中心的初级保健的五个特性评级：可达性／可用性、连续性、综合性、病人参与和医患沟通。十分之一的患者按每个特性从一到四的重要性等级排名，十分之九的患者按所接受护理的体验评分。我们这样计算改善的可能性：负面病人体验比例乘以每个国家重要性平均值。改善可能性分数分为低、中、高等。在改善分数和初级保健结构的三个维度（治理、经济条件和人力发展）

之间进行两两相关分析。

结果 在 26 个国家，初级保健的一个或多个特性有中或高的改善可能性。在 34 个国家中有 23 个国家的护理综合性有中到高等的改善可能性。在所有国家中，医患沟通改善可能性较低。初级保健整体更强的结构与较低的护理连续性和综合性改善可能性相关。在初级保健治理更强的国家，患者认为不太可能改善医疗服务的连续性。初级护理经济条件更好的国家提高所有特性的人为中心护理的可能性更低。

结论 在初级保健结构更强的国家，病人能意识到的初级保健改善可能性更低。

Résumé

Évaluer le potentiel d'amélioration des soins de santé primaires dans 34 pays: une enquête transversale

Objectif Examiner la perception des patients quant au potentiel d'amélioration des soins de santé primaires dans 34 pays.

Méthodes Nous avons mené une enquête transversale sur 69 201 patients qui venaient juste de consulter des médecins

généralistes dans des établissements de soins de santé primaires. Les patients ont évalué cinq caractéristiques des soins de santé primaires axés sur la personne: accessibilité/disponibilité, continuité, exhaustivité, implication du patient et communication entre le médecin et le

Willemijn LA Schäfer et al.

patient. Un dixième des patients ont classé l'importance de chaque caractéristique sur une échelle allant d'un à quatre, et neuf dixièmes ont noté leur expérience des soins reçus. Nous avons calculé le potentiel d'amélioration en multipliant la proportion d'expériences négatives des patients avec le score moyen d'importance danschaque pays. Les scores ont été répartis en potentiels d'amélioration faible, moyen et élevé. Nous avons effectué des corrélations par paire entre les scores d'amélioration et les trois dimensions de la structure des soins de santé primaires: gouvernance, conditions économiques et constitution de la main-d'œuvre.

Résultats Dans 26 pays, une ou plusieurs caractéristiques des soins de santé primaires présentaient des potentiels d'amélioration moyen ou élevé. L'exhaustivité des soins avait un potentiel d'amélioration moyen

à élevé dans 23 des 34 pays. Dans tous les pays, la communication entre le médecin et le patient présentait un potentiel d'amélioration faible. Une structure globale plus forte des soins de santé primaires était corrélée avec un potentiel plus faible d'amélioration pour la continuité et l'exhaustivité des soins. Dans les pays avec une gouvernance plus forte des soins de santé primaires, les patients percevaient un moindre potentiel pour améliorer la continuité des soins. Les pays présentant de meilleures conditions économiques pour les soins de santé primaires avaient un moindre potentiel pour l'amélioration de toutes les caractéristiques des soins de santé axés sur la personne.

Conclusion Dans les pays avec une structure plus forte des soins de santé primaires, les patients perçoivent un moindre potentiel d'amélioration pour les soins de santé primaires.

Резюме

Оценка потенциала улучшения первичной медицинской помощи в 34 странах: перекрестное исследование

Цель Исследовать восприятие пациентами потенциала улучшения первичной медицинской помощи в 34 странах.

Методы Было проведено перекрестное исследование 69 201 пациента, которые посещали только терапевтов в учреждениях первичной медицинской помощи. Пациенты дали оценку пяти характеристикам целенаправленной первичной медицинской помощи: доступность/наличие, непрерывность, комплексность, участие пациента и коммуникация между врачом и пациентом. Одна десятая пациентов расположила по важности каждую характеристику на шкале от одного до четырех, а девять десятых пациентов оценили свой опыт получения медицинской помощи. Потенциал улучшения рассчитывался путем умножения части пациентов с отрицательным опытом на средний балл важности в каждой стране. Баллы делились на низкий, средний и высокий потенциал улучшения. Попарные корреляции выводились между баллами улучшения и тремя характеристиками структуры первичной медицинской помощи: руководством, экономическим положением и подготовкой трудовых ресурсов.

Результаты В 26 странах одна или более характеристик первичной медицинской помощи обладали средним или высоким потенциалом улучшения. Комплексность медицинской помощи обладала потенциалом улучшения от среднего до высокого в 23 из 34 стран. Во всех странах коммуникация между врачом и пациентом имела низкий потенциал улучшения. В целом сильная структура первичной медицинской помощи была связана с низким потенциалом улучшения непрерывности и комплексности медицинской помощи. В странах с эффективным руководством первичной медицинской помощью пациенты усматривали меньший потенциал для улучшения непрерывности медицинской помощи. Страны с лучшим экономическим положением в первичной медицинской помощи обладали меньшим потенциалом улучшения всех характеристик целенаправленной помощи пациенту.

Вывод В странах с эффективной структурой первичной медицинской помощи пациенты усматривали меньший потенциал улучшения в данной области.

Resumen

Evaluación del potencial de mejora de la atención primaria en 34 países: un estudio transversal

Objetivo Investigar las percepciones de los pacientes acerca de la mejora en la atención primaria en 34 países.

Métodos Se realizó una encuesta transversal de 69 201 pacientes que acababan de visitar médicos generales en centros de atención primaria. Los pacientes evaluaron cinco características de la atención primaria centrada en la persona: accesibilidad y disponibilidad, continuidad, exhaustividad, implicación del paciente, así como comunicación entre médico y paciente. Una décima parte de los pacientes clasificó la importancia de cada característica en una escala de uno a cuatro y nueve de cada diez pacientes evaluaron sus experiencias de la atención recibida. Se calculó el potencial de mejora multiplicando la proporción de experiencias negativas de pacientes con la puntuación media de la importancia en cada país. Las puntuaciones se dividieron en potencial de mejora bajo, medio y alto. Se realizaron correlaciones por pares entre las puntuaciones de mejora y las tres dimensiones de la estructura de atención primaria, a saber, gestión, condiciones económicas y desarrollo laboral.

Resultados En 26 países, una o más características de la atención primaria tenían potenciales de mejora medios o altos. El carácter integral de la atención tenía un potencial de mejora entre medio y alto en 23 de 34 países. En todos los países, la comunicación entre médico y paciente tenía un potencial de mejora bajo. Una estructura global más fuerte de la atención primaria se correlacionó con un menor potencial de mejora en la continuidad y exhaustividad de la atención. En los países con una política de dirección de la atención primaria más sólida, los pacientes percibieron un potencial menor de mejora de la continuidad de la atención. Los países con mejores condiciones económicas para la atención primaria presentaron un potencial menor para la mejora de todas las características de la atención centradas en la persona.

Conclusión En países con una estructura de atención primaria más sólida, los pacientes perciben un menor potencial de mejora de la atención primaria.

References

1. Starfield B. Is patient-centered care the same as person-focused care? Perm J. 2011 Spring;15(2):63–9. doi: http://dx.doi.org/10.7812/TPP/10-148 PMID: 21841928

2. De Maeseneer J, van Weel C, Daeren L, Leyns C, Decat P, Boeckxstaens P, et al. From "patient" to "person" to "people": the need for integrated, people-centered healthcare. Int J Pers Cent Med. 2012;2(3):601–14.

3. van Campen C, Sixma HJ, Kerssens JJ, Peters L, Rasker JJ. Assessing patients' priorities and perceptions of the quality of health care: the development of the QUOTE-Rheumatic-Patients instrument. Br J Rheumatol. 1998 Apr;37(4):362–8. doi: http://dx.doi.org/10.1093/rheumatology/37.4.362 PMID: 9619883

4. Sixma HJ, van Campen C, Kerssens JJ, Peters L. Quality of care from the perspective of elderly people: the QUOTE-elderly instrument. Age Ageing. 2000 Mar;29(2):173–8. doi: http://dx.doi.org/10.1093/ageing/29.2.173 PMID: 10791453

5. Sixma HJ, Kerssens JJ, Campen CV, Peters L. Quality of care from the patients' perspective: from theoretical concept to a new measuring instrument. Health Expect. 1998 Nov;1(2):82–95. doi: http://dx.doi.org/10.1046/j.1369-6513.1998.00004.x PMID: 11281863

6. Groenewegen PP, Kerssens JJ, Sixma HJ, van der Eijk I, Boerma WG. What is important in evaluating health care quality? An international comparison of user views. BMC Health Serv Res. 2005 Feb 21;5(1):16. doi: http://dx.doi.org/10.1186/1472-6963-5-16 PMID: 15723701

7. Kerssens JJ, Groenewegen PP, Sixma HJ, Boerma WG, van der Eijk I. Comparison of patient evaluations of health care quality in relation to WHO measures of achievement in 12 European countries. Bull World Health Organ. 2004 Feb;82(2):106–14. PMID: 15042232

8. Grol R, Wensing M, Mainz J, Ferreira P, Hearnshaw H, Hjortdahl P, et al. Patients' priorities with respect to general practice care: an international comparison. European Task Force on Patient Evaluations of General Practice (EUROPEP). Fam Pract. 1999 Feb;16(1):4–11. doi: http://dx.doi.org/10.1093/fampra/16.1.4 PMID: 10321388

9. Jung H, Wensing M, de Wilt A, Olesen F, Grol R. Comparison of patients' preferences and evaluations regarding aspects of general practice care. Fam Pract. 2000 Jun;17(3):236–42. doi: http://dx.doi.org/10.1093/fampra/17.3.236 PMID: 10846142

10. The world health report 2008: primary health care now more than ever. Geneva: World Health Organization; 2008.

11. Kringos D, Boerma W, Bourgueil Y, Cartier T, Dedeu T, Hasvold T, et al. The strength of primary care in Europe: an international comparative study. Br J Gen Pract. 2013 Nov;63(616):e742–50. doi: http://dx.doi.org/10.3399/bjgp13X674422 PMID: 24267857

12. Kringos DS, Boerma WG, Hutchinson A, van der Zee J, Groenewegen PP. The breadth of primary care: a systematic literature review of its core dimensions. BMC Health Serv Res. 2010;10(1):65. doi: http://dx.doi.org/10.1186/1472-6963-10-65 PMID: 20226084

13. Kringos DS. The importance of measuring and improving the strength of primary care in Europe: results of an international comparative study. Türk Aile Hek Derg. 2013;17(4):14.

14. Schäfer WLA, Boerma WG, Kringos DS, De Maeseneer J, Gress S, Heinemann S, et al. QUALICOPC, a multi-country study evaluating quality, costs and equity in primary care. BMC Fam Pract. 2011;12(1):115. doi: http://dx.doi.org/10.1186/1471-2296-12-115 PMID: 22014310

15. Schäfer WL, Boerma WG, Kringos DS, De Ryck E, Greß S, Heinemann S, et al. Measures of quality, costs and equity in primary health care instruments developed to analyse and compare primary care in 35 countries. Qual Prim Care. 2013;21(2):67–79. PMID: 23735688

16. Delnoij DM, Rademakers JJ, Groenewegen PP. The Dutch consumer quality index: an example of stakeholder involvement in indicator development. BMC Health Serv Res. 2010;10(1):88. doi: http://dx.doi.org/10.1186/1472-6963-10-88 PMID: 20370925

17. Meuwissen LE, de Bakker DH. 'Consumer quality'-index General practice care' measures patients' experiences and compares general practices with each other. Ned Tijdschr Geneeskd. 2009;153:A180. [Dutch]. PMID: 19900331

18. Kringos DS, Boerma WG, Bourgueil Y, Cartier T, Hasvold T, Hutchinson A, et al. The European primary care monitor: structure, process and outcome indicators. BMC Fam Pract. 2010;11(1):81. doi: http://dx.doi.org/10.1186/1471-2296-11-81 PMID: 20979612

19. Noordman J, Koopmans B, Korevaar JC, van der Weijden T, van Dulmen S. Exploring lifestyle counselling in routine primary care consultations: the professionals' role. Fam Pract. 2013 Jun;30(3):332–40. doi: http://dx.doi.org/10.1093/fampra/cms077 PMID: 23221102

20. Noordman J. Lifestyle counselling by physicians and practice nurses in primary care: an analysis of daily practice [Dissertation]. Nijmegen: Radboud University; 2013.

21. Grol R, Wensing M, Mainz J, Jung HP, Ferreira P, Hearnshaw H, et al.; European Task Force on Patient Evaluations of General Practice Care (EUROPEP). Patients in Europe evaluate general practice care: an international comparison. Br J Gen Pract. 2000 Nov;50(460):882–7. PMID: 11141874

22. van den Brink-Muinen A, Verhaak PF, Bensing JM, Bahrs O, Deveugele M, Gask L, et al. Doctor-patient communication in different European health care systems: relevance and performance from the patients' perspective. Patient Educ Couns. 2000 Jan;39(1):115–27. doi: http://dx.doi.org/10.1016/S0738-3991(99)00098-1 PMID: 11013553

23. Patient experience 2011/12: key findings of the New Zealand health survey. Wellington: Ministry of Health; 2013.

24. Healthy communities: Australians' experiences with primary health care in 2010-11. Sydney: National Health Performance Authority; 2013.

25. Laberge M, Pang J, Walker K, Wong S, Hogg W, Wodchis W, et al. QUALICOPC (Quality and Costs of Primary Care) Canada: a focus on the aspects of primary care most highly rated by current patients of primary care practices. Ottawa: Canadian Foundation for Healthcare Improvement; 2014.

26. Hogg W, Dyke E. Improving measurement of primary care system performance. Can Fam Physician. 2011 Jul;57(7):758–60, e241–3. PMID: 21753091

27. Blendon RJ, Schoen C, DesRoches C, Osborn R, Zapert K. Common concerns amid diverse systems: health care experiences in five countries. Health Aff (Millwood). 2003 May-Jun;22(3):106–21. doi: http://dx.doi.org/10.1377/hlthaff.22.3.106 PMID: 12757276

28. Schoen C, Osborn R, Huynh PT, Doty M, Zapert K, Peugh J, et al. Taking the pulse of health care systems: experiences of patients with health problems in six countries. Health Aff (Millwood). 2005 Jul-Dec;Suppl Web Exclusives:W5-509–25. PMID: 16269444

Attribution

Schäfer WLA, Boerma WGW, Murante AM, Sixma HJM, Schellevis FG, Groenewegen PP. Assessing the potential for improvement of primary care in 34 countries: A cross-sectional survey. *Bulletin of the World Health Organization* 2015;93:161–168. doi: http://dx.doi.org/10.2471/BLT.14.140368. Reproduced with permission.

CHAPTER 9

Ibero-America

*Juan Victor Ariel Franco, Lidia Caballero
and Mauricio Alberto Rodríguez Escobar*

Health systems and primary care teams in the Latin American Region
Summary of the WONCA-CIMF Panel in Lima

Juan Victor Ariel Franco, Lidia Caballero
and Mauricio Alberto Rodríguez Escobar

INTRODUCTION

The Alma-Ata Declaration of 1978 defined the components of primary health care (PHC) and highlighted their role in health systems. PHC is an efficient way to reach the UN Sustainable Development Goals and not only in the 'Good health and well-being' area, since, for example, the active participation of the community, defined within PHC, is a key element in all areas of development.

Many challenges to the PHC strategy have emerged with its variable implementation across the world. The interaction between health systems and PHC is complex considering the multiple stakeholders defining health policies in each region. Latin America is composed primarily of lower and middle-income countries (LMIC), with relatively young democracies that have suffered, in many cases, civilian and/or military coup d'états and economic crises. While culturally diverse, Latin America is traversed by a common identity and history. See Table 9.1 for some key features of the region.

WONCA-CIMF 2017 PANEL

For this article, we invited representatives from Latin American countries associated with WONCA-CIMF to a panel that was presented at the Ibero-American Confederation of Family Medicine (CIMF) Conference in Lima, Peru, which took

TABLE 9.1   Key Features of the Latin American Region

Population	639 million people
Gross domestic product per capita (range)	US$ 25,564 (Chile) to US$ 1,794 (Haiti)
Language (as first language)	Spanish 60%, Portuguese 34%, Other 6%
Religion	Christianism 90% (mostly Catholic)
Literacy rate	Over 94% for most countries
Human development index (range)	0.847 (Chile) – 0.493 (Haiti)

place in August 2017. For this panel, the participants were asked to reply to four key questions regarding PHC in the region: What are the most important problems for PHC implementation? Are some of these problems common in the Latin American Region? What are the successful models of PHC implementation? What is the role of scientific societies like WONCA-CIMF? We also asked the participants to describe their health systems, how PHC is structured and how PHC teams are composed, the relationship between PHC and other community services and the impact of PHC in each country.

In this article, we will summarize the responses of those participants together with the online discussion that followed the panel presentation, highlighting some country-specific aspects of this topic.

HEALTH SYSTEMS IN THE REGION

There is a wide variety of structures of health systems in the region. In most countries, there is an overlap of subsystems involving social security, private health care and the public sector. The social security sector represents those individuals who receive health care from their contributions through their salary. The private sector involves private hospitals, health care maintenance organizations (HMOs) and other providers that not only provide health care to those privately insured but also to those in social security and the public sector.

ARGENTINA

Argentina is divided into 23 provinces, and its Constitution defines a democratic federal government. This federal system has posed barriers to the implementation of a unified health system based on the PHC strategy, to which this country adhered in 1978 (Alma-Ata Declaration). The poor articulation of health and fiscal policies by the provincial governments and the national government provides a scenario in which PHC has been applied inconsistently. At the same time, other stakeholders have taken a leading role in the organization of health systems: social security (financed by the contributions from employees and managed by unions) and private medicine. During the last 40 years, health care systems have focused on hospital-based and specialized care, and private medical providers have proliferated to the detriment of the public providers. Additionally, social security, private medicine and public health care subsystems have wide overlap and little coordination.

Another problem for the PHC strategy is the shortage of professionals trained in primary care. The available offers are not attractive to applicants, and in many cases there are vacancies. Taking as an example the specialists in family and general medicine, in the year 2015 only 39% of training positions were covered and the postulant/positions ratio was 0.57. As a reference, we could mention that other clinical specialties such as paediatrics and internal medicine have a applicants/positions ratio >2 and 76% of the positions were covered.

Some strategies have been implemented for the integration of PHC teams in vertical government programmes for specific diseases. The widest implementation of a universal health care strategy was the 'Plan Nacer' (2004, initially planned for children), later called 'Plan Sumar' (2012, expanded to pregnant women, adolescents and individuals aged up to 64 years old). These pay for performance (P4P) plans financed PHC teams to provide health care at the point of care based on several indicators, mostly related to PHC interventions. A reduction in growth stunting in children has been documented after the implementation of this plan. The impact on other health outcomes remains uncertain.

ECUADOR

There are several subsystems in this country that are articulated through the Interinstitutional Public Health Network. Nevertheless, the variability of clinical and administrative management generates differences in health care for the end user. Access to health care has important gaps, so that universalization has not been a success. There were several attempts at organizing a universal health care coverage strategy, but in most cases, it made explicit guarantees for pregnant women and children. The 2008 reform of the Constitution stated that health is a right and instituted the National System of Social Inclusion and Equity, guaranteeing the access to free, universal, progressive and equitable health care. In the same year, the New Model for Integrated Care in Family, Community and Intercultural Health was established, which established an organization of health care and the financing mechanisms for the adequate implementation of PHC.

Ecuador also established a National Postgraduate in Family and Community Medicine, which is one of the most important strategies related to the first level of care and PHC; however, the current model does not provide a structure in which the family physician can exert their full capacity due to the limited time in consultation, the excessive bureaucracy, the lack of actual regulations organizing the different levels of care and the limited offer of continued medical education.

MEXICO

Health is protected by the Mexican Constitution. The health system is highly fragmented in the public and private sector with a lack of intersectoral coordination. Social security covers less than half of the population, representing the formal working sectors. Popular health insurance covers almost the other half of the population from the lower income sectors; however, a significant number of Mexicans do not have health coverage. Popular health insurance raised a measure to achieve universal health coverage, facilitating access to prenatal care and other preventive services, as well as chronic care conditions management and catastrophic health care expenditures. This initiative, while praised by those claiming reductions in morbidity and mortality associated with health care inequities, has received criticism from its narrow scope when covering PHC conditions, since most of the popular health insurance is delivered through vertical programmes ('The Doctor in Your Home', 'Home Care of the Chronic Patient', 'Health Caravans'). Additionally, some have argued that the interventions in public health are usually poorly contextualized. Most of the care in this country remains hospital-based and PHC teams lack the resources to provide effective care.

The interest in family medicine as a medical specialty has declined over the years, with a decreasing number of applicants. The centralized residency programme available at the National Autonomous University of Mexico (UNAM) has a three-year programme, half of which is hospital-based. This prospect reduces the human resource availability in PHC.

PANAMA

Health care in this country is administered by the Ministry of Health and social security, providing coverage to 84% of the population; however, there is great overlap in the financing of health care resources for which there are plans to create a national health plan. PHC teams usually involve many disciplines, but they are relatively understaffed in critical specialties such as nurses and family physicians. The system includes many 'sanitary stations', in which health care is not provided by certified health care professionals. The Ministry of Health has been making efforts to provide a better distribution of professionals and resources to local PHC effectors.

Some of PHC services are framed in vertical programmes such as 'Care for the Elderly' or 'Domiciliary Care for Chronic Patients', but they are not necessarily linked to PHC teams. An attempt to integrate PHC was developed in the Integrated Health Services Network, including reference and counter-reference tools to link different levels of care; however, its implementation might be incomplete.

COLOMBIA

In Colombia, the reforms in the health system towards primary health care have been relatively recent. Law 100 of 1993 promulgated a system to achieve universal health coverage with a large participation of private insurers. The provision of services is public and private and financed with public money. This reform has resulted in an increase in the coverage of the insured population, which increased from 15.7% in 1990 to 96.6% in 2014. However, access and equity limitations have been reported, with significant differences between regions and between urban and rural populations. Vertical programmes addressing specific conditions, such as diabetes have been implemented to deliver some PHC services for chronic diseases and prevention. There are difficulties in the articulation of collective and individual actions and in the establishment of integrated health networks. There was an attempt to improve this with the promulgation of Law 1438 in 2011; however, the complexity of articulating a public or collective health system with a geographic territorial distribution and a referenced population has caused difficulties when implementing what the law proposed. Law 1751 of 2015 guarantees the right to health, and Resolution 429 of 2017 establishes the Policy of Comprehensive Health Care, which defines a Model of Comprehensive Health Care. They are still in the planning stage and have not been implemented.

There have been attempts at training human resources for PHC. A unique programme of specialization in family medicine has been established for physicians and a specialization programme in family health for other professionals, which seeks better interdisciplinary teams of primary health care. The proportion of specialists in family medicine compared to the total number of physicians is 0.7%. In 2010, there were 0.37 nurses per doctor and 1.67 doctors per 1,000 inhabitants. There is a shortage of human resources in health in many rural areas, with problems of human resource distribution. This may impede PHC teams when attempting to achieve resolutions of common health problems in the first level of care.

PARAGUAY

Health is provided by the public and private sectors with a wide overlap and fragmentation. The Constitution establishes the right to health care; however, it is estimated that 35% of Paraguayans do not have health coverage. In Paraguay, the concept of PHC is limited to the Family Health Units (FHU), a system implemented in 2008 to widen services to achieve universal health coverage. However, 90% of physicians who work in PHC do not have a specialty, and family medicine specialists do not receive incentives for their qualifications. The current 800 FHUs cover a little more than 30% of the population, and many of these FHUs are incomplete (either lacking a doctor, nurses or community agents). It is estimated that an additional 1,000 FHUs (about 1,800 in total) are necessary to achieve full coverage for communities requiring the care of PHC teams.

DOMINICAN REPUBLIC

The Laws 42-01 and 87-01 (2001) established the right to health care in this country by means of social security or the National Health System (public sector). Social security comprises the Health Family Insurance, which is divided into a contributive regime (for formal workers) and a state-subsidized regime. However, more than half of Dominicans are outside this system and rely on the National Health System, which provides health care at a cost for individuals. This system is organized in PHC and specialized care (secondary and tertiary care). PHC units are proposed to deliver all the functions related to primary care in terms of prevention and resolution of common problems in health. Nevertheless, they are usually understaffed, staffed by health care professionals without PHC training (e.g. doctors without speciality) and do not have sufficient resources to deal with the population's needs. It is estimated that an additional 700 over the existing 1,725 PHC units are required to meet the needs of the 10 million Dominicans.

COMMON CHALLENGES IN THE REGION

The representatives for each country have expressed common concerns related to the fragmentation and overlap of the organizations and structures involved in the governance, financing and delivery of care. The private sector has grown in the region, providing health care not only to those privately insured but also to those affiliated with many of the government-sponsored programmes to make explicit guarantees for health care to achieve universal health care coverage. This complex landscape creates difficulties in governance. Nevertheless, some alliances with international organizations, such as the Pan American Health Organization (PAHO)/World Health Organization (WHO), have made it possible for some countries to establish policies to ensure more equitable care and a focus on PHC.

Another common problem in the region is the insufficient human resources for primary care, in the form of trained nurses and primary care physicians. This phenomenon has multifactorial roots, some of them related to the pre-eminence of specialized care, in which primary care specialities are not attractive to young health care practitioners. The endorsement of universities and governments in the placement of family and community medicine postgraduate programmes sound promising, but the widespread dissemination of these programmes have not guaranteed the placement of physicians in these positions. WONCA-CIMF has been working throughout these years in the empowerment and leadership of local family medicine programmes in each country, promoting continued medical education activities.

Only a few of the countries in the WONCA-CIMF region participated in this panel, which could represent a limitation of this document. In Table 9.2 we have listed the countries that are members of WONCA-CIMF whose health care system data we could retrieve. For this reason, we would like to mention that two countries of this region have developed initiatives to promote PHC: Spain and Brazil. Spain's modern national health care system was created in 1986; it is financed by the state, administrated by each autonomous region and organized in different levels of care.

TABLE 9.2 CIMF Countries Categorized According to Their Health System

Country	Free Health Care	Universal Health Care
Argentina*	Free	Universal
Bolivia	Not Free	Not Universal
Brazil	Free	Universal
Chile	Free	Universal
Colombia*	Free	Universal
Costa Rica*	Free	Universal
Cuba	Free	Universal
Dominican Republic*	Not Free	Not Universal
Ecuador*	Free	Universal
El Salvador	Free	Not Universal
Mexico*	Free	Universal
Nicaragua	Free	Not Universal
Panama	Free	Not Universal
Paraguay*	Free	Universal
Peru	Free	Universal
Puerto Rico	N/A	N/A
Portugal	Free	Universal
Spain	Free	Universal
Uruguay	Free	Universal
Venezuela	Free	Universal

Note: **CIMF:** Ibero-American Confederation of Family Medicine (*) Countries that participated in the Panel. **N/A:** not available. **Free Health Care:** refers to a publicly funded health care that provides primary services free of charge or for a nominal fee to all its citizens, with no exclusions based on income or wealth. **Universal Health Care:** usually refers to a health care system that provides health care and financial protection to more than 90% of the citizens of a country. This information on care was taken from: http://globalresidenceindex.com/hnwi-index/health-index/ (last accessed March 2018) based on information provided by the government websites, WHO and Pacific Prime Insurance.

PHC is delivered by diverse teams in the multiple PHC units across the country. The training of family physicians is guaranteed by 1,810 residency vacancies per year. Nevertheless, Spain also is traversed by the common problems in health systems worldwide, such as the increased costs in health expenditure, a renovated criticism of the quality of PHC delivery, and the aversion of doctors when choosing family medicine as a speciality. Brazil implemented a Family Health Programme in 1994 as an effective way to deliver PHC in their community; it was renewed and elevated in hierarchy in 2006 as a Family Health Strategy. This was possible thanks to the strategic allocation of funds for PHC teams distributed across the country and working in collaboration as networks of health care delivery. PHC professionals include people from different disciplines, including over 350,000 community health workers. This programme has been shown to reduce child mortality, cardiovascular disease morbidity and hospitalizations, among other outcomes.

CONCLUSIONS

We expect this document to reflect the common challenges that our health systems faced when implementing primary health care in the region. We acknowledge that we had some local successes, such as in the case of Brazil and Spain, but we need to reflect on the remaining difficulties for the wide dissemination of primary care. We believe that there is room for organizations like WONCA-CIMF to partner with international organizations, such as PAHO/WHO, and individual countries to design actions to overcome these difficulties related to policy development and training of high-quality human resources for primary care. Additionally, many of the issues related to the access and development of primary care may also relate to the high socio-economic inequity in the region, which might require intersectoral strategies with other areas of local and regional government.

ABOUT THE AUTHORS

Juan Victor Ariel Franco (Federación Argentina de Medicina Familiar y General [FAMFyG] – Argentina; Servicio de Medicina Familiar y Comunitaria – Hospital Italiano de Buenos Aires – Argentina)

Lidia Caballero (Federación Argentina de Medicina Familiar y General [FAMFyG] – Argentina; Hospital Dr. Pedro Baliña – Posadas, Misiones – Argentina)

Mauricio Alberto Rodríguez Escobar (Colombian Society of Family Medicine – Colombia)

Contributors: Matías Tonnelier (Argentina), Fausto Gady Torres Toala (Ecuador), Homero de los Santos Reséndiz (México), Patricia Rivera (Panama), Yokasta Germosén Almonte (Republica Domincana), Diana Yuruhán (Paraguay), Andres Szwako (Paraguay)

CHAPTER 10

North America: Canada

Brian Hutchison and Richard Glazier

PRIMARY CARE

By Brian Hutchison and Richard Glazier

Ontario's Primary Care Reforms Have Transformed The Local Care Landscape, But A Plan Is Needed For Ongoing Improvement

DOI: 10.1377/hlthaff.2012.1087
HEALTH AFFAIRS 32,
NO. 4 (2013): –
©2013 Project HOPE—
The People-to-People Health
Foundation, Inc

ABSTRACT Primary care in Ontario, Canada, has undergone a series of reforms designed to improve access to care, patient and provider satisfaction, care quality, and health system efficiency and sustainability. We highlight key features of the reforms, which included patient enrollment with a primary care provider; funding for interprofessional primary care organizations; and physician reimbursement based on varying blends of fee-for-service, capitation, and pay-for-performance. With nearly 75 percent of Ontario's population now enrolled in these new models, total payments to primary care physicians increased by 32 percent between 2006 and 2010, and the proportion of Ontario primary care physicians who reported overall satisfaction with the practice of medicine rose from 76 percent in 2009 to 84 percent in 2012. However, primary care in Ontario also faces challenges. There is no meaningful performance measurement system that tracks the impact of these innovations, for example. A better system of risk adjustment is also needed in capitated plans so that groups have the incentive to take on high-need patients. Ongoing investment in these models is required despite fiscal constraints. We recommend a clearly articulated policy road map to continue the transformation.

Brian Hutchison (hutchb@ mcmaster.ca) is a professor emeritus in the Department of Family Medicine and the Department of Clinical Epidemiology and Biostatistics at McMaster University and senior adviser for primary care to Health Quality Ontario, in Toronto.

Richard Glazier is a senior scientist and program lead of primary care and population health at the Institute for Clinical Evaluative Sciences, in Toronto, Ontario.

Canada's ten provincial and three territorial health systems operate within a national legislative framework, the Canada Health Act of 1984. Under the act, provinces and territories receive health care funding to provide universal, public, first-dollar coverage of medically necessary physician and hospital services. Because the act requires coverage of only physician and hospital services, the extent of public coverage of other health services, such as prescription drugs, vision care, home care, and long-term care, varies among the provinces and territories.

In 2010, 71 percent of Canada's health spending was publicly funded.[1] However, Canada's health care delivery system is largely private.

Most physicians are independent contractors who are reimbursed by the provincial or territorial health plan on a fee-for-service basis. Almost all hospitals are owned and operated by private not-for-profit entities.

With more than thirteen million residents, Ontario is Canada's most populous province. Historically, primary care in Ontario was delivered predominantly by solo and small-group practices owned and managed by physicians. Physicians are paid by the Ontario Ministry of Health and Long-Term Care and may not bill patients or third parties for services covered by the public health insurance plan. Ontario has the second-lowest ratio of primary care physicians to population among Canada's ten provinces: 92 per 100,000.[2]

Canada's Health System Performance

During the 1980s and 1990s many industrialized countries invested heavily in strengthening primary care. Canada did not, and its primary care infrastructure and patient access to primary care suffered. A recent survey of primary care physicians in ten wealthy industrialized countries[3] showed that Canadian physicians ranked second-lowest on use of electronic medical records; were least likely to offer online appointment scheduling or to respond via e-mail to patients' medical questions or concerns; and were less likely than primary care physicians in all but one other country to work with nurses, therapists, or other nonphysician clinicians.

In the early 2000s a new policy environment emerged in Canada in response to an improved fiscal climate, growing public and professional dissatisfaction with the country's primary care status quo, and national reviews[4,5] that highlighted the importance of primary care to overall health system performance. Policy makers began to embrace a gradual approach to reforming primary care.[6,7]

Five national reform objectives were established. These were increasing access to primary care organizations that would provide a defined set of services to a defined population; increasing emphasis on health promotion, disease and injury prevention, and chronic disease management; expanding all-day, every-day access to essential services; establishing interdisciplinary primary care teams; and facilitating coordination and integration with other health services. To pay for the reforms, the federal government committed substantial funds to advancing primary health care, home care, and catastrophic prescription drug coverage.

Ontario's Primary Care Reform Strategy

Ontario moved swiftly to develop a variety of new care delivery and payment models[8] that were responsive to the new national goals. The Ministry of Health and Long-Term Care worked closely with major stakeholders, including physician groups such as the Ontario Medical Association, to develop diverse primary care models that were voluntary for both providers and patients. From 2002 to 2007 a number of new primary care organizational and funding models were initiated, having different characteristics to suit diverse provider and patient communities (Exhibit 1). These models are described more fully in the online Appendix.[9]

Voluntary participation by patients and providers in these new models of care provided opportunities for those ready to embrace innovation to do so without requiring universal participation or adoption. Physicians were attracted to the new models by the promise of increased income under the new arrangements;[10] improved infrastructure, such as electronic medical records; additional clinical and administrative staffing; sharing of after-hours on-call work; and the positive experience reported by early adopters. Patients readily accepted the new models because they preserved the continuity of physician-patient relationships.

Key Policy Initiatives

Since 2000 Ontario has pursued three major, interconnected policy initiatives: new physician reimbursement and organizational models, patient enrollment with a primary care provider, and support for interprofessional team-based care.[8]

NEW MODELS Physicians practicing in the new organization and payment models are reimbursed through various blends of payment types, including capitation, which is payment per patient per month; fee-for-service; salary; and pay-for-performance.

In two of the reimbursement models, the Family Health Organization and the Family Health Network, capitation is the principal component. Capitation payments are adjusted for the age and sex of enrolled patients. In 2012, 39 percent of Ontario's family physicians participated in these models. In two other models, Family Health Group and Comprehensive Care, fee-for-service is the main element. Twenty-nine percent of Ontario's family physicians participated in these two models in 2012.

Physicians working in Community Health Centres, described below, are salaried employees. In two additional models, the Rural and Northern Physician Group Agreement and the model for physicians working in community-governed Family Health Teams, reimbursement is salary based with additional incentive payments. Physicians working in Family Health Teams with physician governance or mixed community and physician governance are paid through one of three remuneration models: Family Health Organization, Family Health Network, or Rural and Northern Physician Group Agreement.

All blended reimbursement models include special fees or premiums, which vary across models, for providing priority services such as reproductive care, palliative care, and home visits. They also include graduated pay-for-performance for achieving specified levels of preventive care coverage among enrolled patients and incentive fees for the management

EXHIBIT 1

Primary Care Organizational And Funding Models In Ontario

Characteristic	Community Health Centre (1979)	Family Health Network (2002)	Family Health Group (2003)	Rural and Northern Physician Group Agreement (2004)	Comprehensive Care Model (2005)	Family Health Team (2005)	Family Health Organization[a] (2007)
	Model (year introduced)						
Physician reimbursement	Salary	Blended capitation	Blended fee-for-service	Blended salary	Blended fee-for-service	Blended capitation or blended salary	Blended capitation
Targeted financial incentives	No	Yes	Yes	Yes	Yes	Yes	Yes
Formal patient enrollment	No	Yes	Yes	Yes	Yes	Yes	Yes
Minimum group size (physicians)	None	3	3	1	1	3	3
Governance	Community board	Physician-led	Physician-led	Physician-led	Physician-led	Physician-led, community board, or mixed	Physician-led
Interprofessional team members	Yes	Limited	Limited	No	No	Yes	Limited
After-hours care requirements	Yes	Yes	Yes	Yes	Optional	Yes	Yes

SOURCE Ontario Ministry of Health and Long-Term Care. **NOTE** A fuller version of this table is available in the Appendix (Note 9 in text). [a]Created through the harmonization of two preexisting models: Health Service Organizations (introduced in 1978) and Primary Care Networks (introduced in 1999).

of patients with diabetes and congestive heart failure and for smoking cessation.

The introduction of these new organization and remuneration models has transformed the primary care landscape in Ontario. In 2012, 76 percent of Ontario's family physicians participated in one of the new primary care reimbursement models, with the other 24 percent remaining in traditional fee-for-service arrangements. This constitutes a dramatic change from 2002, when 94 percent of Ontario's family physicians were in traditional fee-for-service arrangements and just 6 percent in some other kind of reimbursement arrangement (Exhibit 2).

Of the primary care physicians who continued to be reimbursed through traditional fee-for-service arrangements in 2012, about half were in "focused" or specialized practice—for example, emergency department, psychotherapy, hospital medicine, sports medicine, or long-term care.

With limited exceptions, the new primary care reimbursement models required participating physicians to be **PART** of a group practice or practice network of three or more physicians. Partly as a result, the proportion of Ontario primary care physicians who self-identified as solo practitioners declined from 37.4 percent in 2001 to 24.9 percent in 2010.[11,12] Participating practic-

es were also required to provide a minimum number of weekend and evening office hours that varied by group size. Apart from these requirements, the new reimbursement mechanisms support and reward, but do not require, changes in the organization and delivery of care.

Total payments to primary care physicians increased by 32 percent between fiscal year 2006–07 and fiscal year 2009–10, related in large part to the introduction of new reimbursement models.[13] Additionally, average payments to primary care physicians increased at a higher rate than did payments for specialist physicians.[14] The proportion of Ontario primary care physicians who reported overall satisfaction with the practice of medicine increased from 76 percent in 2009 to 84 percent in 2012.[3,15] More Ontario medical school graduates now choose family medicine as their first choice for postgraduate training compared with ten years ago—a shift from 26 percent in 2003 to a percentage that fluctuated between 34 percent and 39 percent during 2009–11.[16]

PATIENT ENROLLMENT Under Ontario's reformed primary care models, patients are not required to enroll, even if their regular physician participates in one of the reimbursement models and offers enrollment in it. Additionally, physicians cannot refuse to enroll a patient because of

EXHIBIT 2

Distribution Of Ontario Family Physicians, By Payment Model, 2002 And 2012

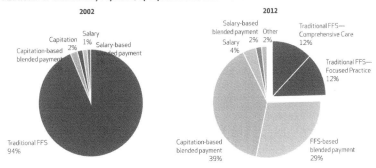

SOURCES Ontario Ministry of Health and Long-Term Care and Institute for Clinical Evaluative Sciences. NOTE FFS is fee-for-service.

the patient's health status or level of need for services. When a patient chooses to enroll with a participating primary care practice, the patient agrees to seek treatment first from the enrolling physician (or group) unless the patient is traveling or experiencing a health emergency. The enrolling physician or group commits to providing comprehensive primary care services to the patient.

Ontario's new primary care practice models are proving popular: The number of patients enrolled with a primary care physician grew from fewer than 600,000 in 2002 to 9.9 million in August 2012, representing 73 percent of the Ontario population (Phil Graham, Ontario Ministry of Health and Long-Term Care, personal communication, August 10, 2012).

PRIMARY CARE TEAMS Expanding interprofessional primary care teams was a key goal of Ontario's primary care reforms. These teams are "groups of professionals from different disciplines who communicate and work together in a formal arrangement to care for a patient population in a primary care setting."[17] They typically include primary care physicians and nurses or nurse practitioners, or both, and a provider from at least one other clinical discipline, such as a social worker, dietitian, or pharmacist. In contrast, traditional primary care practices usually include only physicians, medical office assistants, and—commonly but not always—nurses.

Ontario's emphasis on interprofessional primary care teams is addressed through a network of 75 Community Health Centres, 200 Family Health Teams, and 26 Nurse Practitioner–Led Clinics. The total number of primary care physicians working in interprofessional teams increased from 176 in 2002 to more than 3,000

in 2012 (Graham, personal communication, August 10, 2012, and July 20, 2012). Ontario's Community Health Centres deliver care to socially disadvantaged and hard-to-serve populations and employ almost 400 primary care physicians and more than 300 nurse practitioners.

The province's Family Health Teams serve as patient-centered medical homes, where people can access care from multiple health care providers—most commonly nurses, nurse practitioners, dietitians, mental health workers, social workers, pharmacists, health educators, and occupational therapists—in one setting. They now include more than 2,400 primary care physicians and more than 1,700 other primary health care professionals (Graham, personal communication, July 20, 2012). Ontario's Nurse Practitioner–Led Clinics are similar in concept to Family Health Teams, but in these clinics physicians function mainly in a consulting capacity.

To support the development of interprofessional primary care teams and increase access to primary care, the provincial government has expanded medical, nurse practitioner, and midwifery education programs; increased the number of family medicine residency positions; established educational programs for physician assistants; and expanded the scope of practice of nurse practitioners, midwives, and pharmacists.[18-21] Interprofessional primary care teams now serve close to one-fifth of the province's population.

Additional Initiatives

In addition to the initiatives described above, Ontario embraced other programs to improve access to primary care and strengthen primary care infrastructure.

LINKING UNATTACHED PATIENTS TO A PRIMARY CARE PROVIDER In a further attempt to address the sizable number of Ontarians without a regular primary care provider, the Ministry of Health launched Health Care Connect. This program was designed to help unattached patients obtain a regular primary care provider using nurses known as "care connectors," who attempt to identify a primary care provider willing to accept the patient. A priority focus was patients with high needs for care. Primary care physicians who accepted a high-needs patient received bonus payments for enrolling the patient and also for the patient's first year of care.

By September 2012, 226,371 patients had registered with the program. Of these, 165,328 patients, 16,138 of whom were high-needs, were matched by care connectors with a primary care provider who agreed to accept them as a patient.[22]

FUNDING ADMINISTRATIVE PERSONNEL Except for Community Health Centres, primary care in Ontario has been notable for its lack of administrative infrastructure at the practice level. Family Health Teams are eligible for funding for administrative purposes, including an administrator or executive director. The agreements governing the Family Health Organization and Family Health Network reimbursement models described above allow for "office practice administration" funding to employ an administrator.

ADOPTING ELECTRONIC MEDICAL RECORDS The Ministry of Health has historically subsidized the purchase and implementation of approved clinical management systems, such as electronic medical records, in Family Health Networks and Family Health Organizations and to a lesser extent in other new primary care reimbursement models. However, beginning in 2010 subsidies and technical support were made available to all family physicians, no matter what care model they were a part of. The proportion of Ontario family physicians who reported using an electronic medical record increased from 44 percent in 2009 to 65 percent in 2012.[3,15]

INTEGRATING QUALITY IMPROVEMENT TRAINING AND SUPPORT Efforts to integrate quality improvement methods in Ontario's primary care sector, a recognized need, are ongoing but insufficient given the size of the sector. Learning collaboratives based on the Institute for Healthcare Improvement Breakthrough Series model[23] lead to new hands-on and virtual training that has reached approximately 500 practice-based teams. The Ministry of Health supports this work through Health Quality Ontario, a

ministry-funded government agency.

Challenges And Shortcomings

Despite substantial system-level changes, the impact of Ontario's primary care reforms on processes and outcomes of care is yet to be determined. A time lag in realizing the benefits of policy initiatives is to be expected, particularly for complex innovations such as the implementation of interprofessional teams. Substantial gains in access, quality, or effectiveness of care require reshaping roles and care processes.

However, even at this stage of implementation, several policy shortcomings and missing elements have become apparent. These need to be addressed to ensure that Ontarians reap the full benefit of recent investments in strengthening primary care.

LOCAL PRIMARY CARE GOVERNANCE Ontario's primary care sector continues to be severely fragmented. In all but a few communities, numerous—mainly small—primary care practices and organizations operate independently, lack a common voice, and rarely share resources and expertise. In this environment, effective coordination and integration of primary care with other specialized health and social service sectors is virtually impossible.

Local, appropriately resourced primary care organizations are needed that could assume collective responsibility for clinical performance and service delivery. Such organizations could respond to community needs; negotiate relationships with other health and social services; and coordinate and support the sharing of resources, performance measurement activities, and quality improvement efforts to improve population health.

ONGOING PERFORMANCE MEASUREMENT AND FEEDBACK Ontario lacks a coherent system for ongoing primary care performance measurement and feedback at the practice, organization, and system (community, regional, and provincial) levels. A performance measurement system that taps health administrative data, clinical data from electronic medical records, and patient experience data could regularly provide actionable information to identify strengths and shortcomings, guide service and system planning, and track the impact of policy innovations and quality improvement efforts.

SYSTEMWIDE QUALITY IMPROVEMENT TRAINING AND SUPPORT Several hundred practice-based primary care teams have participated in quality improvement initiatives. However, this number represents a small fraction of the province's primary care practices. A strategy is needed to spread quality improvement training and support across the entire sector, perhaps using provincially supported local primary care organizations as the locus of quality improvement expertise and activity.

Financial incentives targeting improved outcomes will be effective only if primary care providers and managers have the capacity to measure and improve health care processes and outcomes.

IMPROVED ELECTRONIC MEDICAL RECORDS Although the provincial government has made sizable investments in primary care information technology, the current systems have limited interoperability and performance measurement, disease management, and registry capability.

ALIGNMENT OF INCENTIVES WITH HEALTH SYSTEM NEEDS Several elements of current primary care physician payment arrangements require review in light of emerging evidence. Blended payment schemes based on capitation are more conducive to interprofessional team-based care than is fee-for-service remuneration. However, age- and sex-adjusted capitation does not adequately capture the variation in need for primary care services in practices serving sicker, often socially disadvantaged, populations.

Until the capitation-based blended payment rates are risk-adjusted, physicians serving these populations are likely to remain in fee-for-service practice. This reality leaves these providers and their vulnerable patients unable to access the enhanced clinical and administrative resources that are available to those in Family Health Teams, for example, thereby perpetuating and deepening health care inequities. Current evidence indicates that less healthy, low-income, and immigrant Ontarians are underrepresented in the practice populations of capitation-based physicians.[24] Risk-adjusted capitation is needed to address this issue.

Current pay-for-performance incentives also need to be reviewed given their modest or, in some cases, nonexistent impact.[25,26] The "access bonus" component of capitation-based blended payment models is administratively cumbersome; penalizes physicians serving marginalized populations; and, because the access bonus is unaffected by enrolled patients' use of emergency departments, fails to discourage unnecessary emergency department use. This fact may help explain why rates of emergency department visits—after demographics, urban-rural location, and case-mix are controlled for—are higher in the capitation-based models, including Family Health Teams, than in fee-for-service–based models and have not changed appreciably over time.[24,27] Same-day or next-day access to primary care also has not improved

over time.[27]

EFFECTIVE MANAGEMENT OF PERFORMANCE CONTRACTS Contractual agreements between the Ministry of Health and Long-Term Care and physicians participating in patient enrollment models specify the range of services that physicians are required to provide and the terms and conditions under which they must deliver those services. However, contract monitoring has been lax. Not surprisingly, some participating practices have failed to meet their contractual obligations.[13,28]

SYSTEMATIC EVALUATION OF INNOVATION The Ministry of Health frequently commissions evaluations of major policy and health system innovations that identify successes that need to be reinforced and spread and shortcomings that need to be addressed. However, these commissioned evaluations are often inadequately resourced, not subject to scientific review, and begun too late for relevant baseline data to be collected. Moreover, the findings are rarely made public. The results of publicly funded evaluations need to be made publicly available if they are to be effective.

Moving Forward

Many of the continuing needs discussed above are being addressed, at least in part, by the Ministry of Health. For example, a pilot program, Health Links, will support collaborations among primary care providers, specialist physicians, hospitals, home care, and long-term care in nineteen communities to improve care for high-needs patients.[29]

A multistakeholder initiative to develop a comprehensive primary care performance measurement system is under way. The initiative includes the Ministry of Health, data holders, organizations representing primary care providers, patient advocacy groups, and regional health authorities.

Beginning this year, the Ministry of Health will require Family Health Teams, Community Health Centres, and Nurse Practitioner–Led Clinics to prepare and submit annual quality improvement plans to Health Quality Ontario and to report performance measures, including measures of timely access to care.

The latest negotiated agreement between the Ministry of Health and the Ontario Medical Association includes provisions to introduce an "acuity modifier" to address variation in health care need beyond that captured by age and sex adjustment of capitation payments and to review the access bonus. If appropriately designed, the acuity modifier would address the need for risk adjustment of primary care capitation payments identified above. The agreement also includes increased fees and performance incentives for house calls to homebound and frail elderly patients and criteria-based funding for inter-professional health care providers in non–Family Health Team patient enrollment models.[30]

Independent evaluations of Health Quality Ontario's primary care quality improvement collaboratives and learning community are in progress and will be publicly released. A five-year external evaluation of the Family Health Team initiative, commissioned by the Ministry of Health, is in its fourth year. However, the government has not yet committed to making the results public.

Conclusion

The past several years have seen profound changes in the funding and organization of primary care in Ontario. However, budgetary constraints arising from government deficits incurred during the recent recession pose a threat to the ongoing process of transformation, which requires continuing investments. To sustain the transformational momentum, a clearly articulated policy road map that commands the support of the public and key stakeholders is needed. Given the fiscal climate, primary care stakeholders—including the public—will need to mobilize to ensure that Canada's federal and provincial governments stay the course of primary health care renewal. ∎

Support for this research was provided by the Commonwealth Fund. Brian Hutchison has served as a consultant to the Ontario Ministry of Health and Long-Term Care.

NOTES

1 Organization for Economic Cooperation and Development. OECD health data 2012: how does Canada compare [Internet]. Paris: OECD; 2012 [cited 2012 Aug 30]. Available from: http://www.oecd.org/Canada/BriefingNote CANADA2012.pdf

2 Canadian Institute for Health Information. Supply, distribution, and migration of Canadian physicians, 2010. Ottawa (ON): CIHI; 2011.

3 Commonwealth Fund. 2011 Commonwealth Fund International Survey of Primary Care Doctors [Internet]. New York (NY): The Fund; 2012 [cited 2013 Mar 19]. Available from: http://www.commonwealthfund.org/Surveys/2011/Nov/2011-International-Survey.aspx

4 Commission on the Future of Health Care in Canada. Building on values: the future of health care in Canada—final report [Internet]. Saskatoon (SK): Government of Canada; 2002 Nov [cited 2013 Mar 8]. Available from: http://publications.gc.ca/collections/Collection/CP32-85-2002E.pdf

5 Standing Senate Committee on Social Affairs, Science, and Technology. The health of Canadians—federal role—final report. Vol. 6, Recommendations for reform [Internet]. Ottawa (ON); Parliament of Canada; 2002 Oct [cited 2013 Mar 8]. Available from: http://www.parl.gc.ca/Content/SEN/Committee/372/soci/rep/repoct02vol6-e.htm

6 Hutchison B. Primary health care

renewal in Canada: are we nearly there? In: Wilson R, Shortt SED, Dorland J, editors. Implementing primary care reform: barriers and facilitators. Kingston (ON): Queen's University School of Policy Studies; 2004. p. 111–28.

7 Hutchison B. A long time coming: primary healthcare renewal in Canada. Healthc Pap. 2008;8(2):10–24.

8 Hutchison B, Levesque JF, Strumpf E, Coyle N. Primary health care in Canada: systems in motion. Milbank Q. 2011;89(2):256–88.

9 To access the Appendix, click on the Appendix link in the box to the right of the article online.

10 Green ME, Hogg W, Gray D, Manuel D, Koller M, Maaten S, et al. Financial and work satisfaction: impacts of participation in primary care reform on physicians in Ontario. Healthc Policy. 2009;5(2):e161–76.

11 College of Family Physicians of Canada. National Physician Survey 2001, Ontario data. Mississauga (ON): The College; 2002.

12 College of Family Physicians of Canada, Canadian Medical Association, Royal College of Physicians and Surgeons of Canada. National Physician Survey 2010 [Internet]. Mississauga (ON): The College; 2011 [cited 2012 Aug 30]. Table: Provincial results by FP/GP or other specialist, sex, age, and all physicians: Ontario. Available from: http://nationalphysiciansurvey.ca/wp-content/uploads/2012/09/2010-ProvON-Q10a.pdf

13 Office of the Auditor General of

Ontario. 2011 annual report [Internet]. Toronto (ON): The Office; 2012. Chapter 3, Funding alternatives for family physicians; [cited 2013 Mar 19]. Available from: http://www.auditor.on.ca/en/reports_en/en11/306en11.pdf

14 Henry DA, Schultz SE, Glazier RH, Bhatia RS, Dhalla IA, Laupacis A. Payments to Ontario physicians from ministry of health and long-term care sources, 1992/93 to 2009/10: ICES investigative report [Internet]. Toronto (ON): Institute for Clinical Evaluative Sciences; 2012 Feb [cited 2012 May 22]. Available for download from: http://www.ices.on.ca/webpage.cfm?site_id=1&org_id=68

15 Commonwealth Fund. 2009 Commonwealth Fund International Health Policy Survey [Internet]. New York (NY): The Fund; 2009 [cited 2013 Mar 19]. Available from: http://www.commonwealthfund.org/Surveys/2009/Nov/2009-Commonwealth-Fund-International-Health-Policy-Survey.aspx

16 Canadian Resident Matching Service. Reports and statistics—R1 match reports [Internet]. Ottawa (ON): CaRMS; 2003–2011 [cited 2012 Sep 1]. Available for download from: http://www.carms.ca/eng/operations_R1reports_e.shtml

17 Conference Board of Canada. Improving primary health care through collaboration: briefing 1—Current knowledge about interprofessional teams in Canada. Ottawa (ON): The Board; 2012 Oct. p. 2.

18 Ontario Ministry of Health and

PRIMARY CARE

Long-Term Care. Results-based plan briefing book: 2011–12 [Internet]. Toronto (ON): The Ministry; 2012 [cited 2012 Sep 1]. Available from: http://health.gov.on.ca/en/common/ministry/publications/plans/rbp_2011_12.pdf

19 College of Nurses of Ontario. Membership statistics report: 2011 [Internet]. Toronto (ON): CNO; 2012 [cited 2012 Aug 30]. Available from: http://www.cno.org/Global/docs/general/43069_stats/43069_MembershipStatistics2011.pdf

20 College of Midwives of Ontario. Annual report 2010–2011 [Internet]. Toronto (ON): CMO; 2012 [cited 2012 Sep 1]. Available from: http://www.cmo.on.ca/documents/ANNUALREPORT2010-2011FINAL.pdf

21 Government of Ontario [Internet]. Toronto (ON): Government of Ontario; c2012. Press release, Birth centres coming to Ontario; 2012 Mar 20 [cited 2012 Sep 1]. Available from: http://news.ontario.ca/opo/en/2012/03/birth-centres-coming-to-ontario.html

22 Ontario Ministry of Health and Long-Term Care. Public information: Health Care Connect: program results [Internet]. Toronto (ON): The Ministry; 2012 [cited 2013 Feb 6]. Available from: http://health.gov.on.ca/en/ms/healthcareconnect/public/results.aspx

23 Institute for Healthcare Improvement. IHI's collaborative model for achieving breakthrough improvement. Boston (MA): IHI; 2003. (IHI Innovation Series White Paper: The Breakthrough Series).

24 Glazier RH, Kopp A, Schultz S, Kiran T, Henry D. All the right intentions but few of the desired results: lessons on access to primary care from Ontario's patient enrolment models. Healthc Q. 2012;15(3):17–21.

25 Kiran T, Victor JC, Kopp A, Shah BR, Glazier RH. The relationship between financial incentives and quality of diabetes care in Ontario, Canada. Diabetes Care. 2012;35(5):1038–46.

26 Hurley J, DeCicca P, Li J, Buckley G. The response of Ontario primary care physicians to pay-for-performance incentives [Internet]. Hamilton (ON): Centre for Health Economics and Policy Analysis; 2011 Apr 21 [cited 2012 Sep 29]. (CHEPA Working Paper Series, No. 11-02). Available from: http://www.chepa.org/docs/working-papers/11-02.pdf?sfvrsn=2

27 Glazier RH, Zagorski BM, Rayner J. Comparison of primary care models in Ontario by demographics, case mix, and emergency department use, 2008/09 to 2009/10 [Internet]. Toronto (ON): Institute for Clinical Evaluative Sciences; 2012 Mar [cited 2012 May 22]. (ICES Investigative Report). Available from: http://www.ices.on.ca/file/ICES_Primary%20Care%20Models%20English.pdf

28 Howard M, Randall GE. After-hours information given by telephone by family physicians in Ontario. Healthc Policy. 2009;5(2):106–15.

29 Ontario Ministry of Health and Long-Term Care. Ontario's Action Plan for Health Care: making healthy change happen [Internet]. Toronto (ON): The Ministry; 2013 Jan [cited 2013 Mar 11]. Available from: http://www.health.gov.on.ca/en/ms/ecfa/healthy_change/docs/progress_healthychange_en.pdf

30 Ontario Ministry of Health and Long-Term Care. 2012 physician services agreement—primary care changes. Info Bulletin [serial on the Internet]. 2013 Feb 25 [cited 28 Feb 2013]. Available from: http://www.health.gov.on.ca/en/pro/programs/ohip/bulletins/11000/bul11062.pdf

ABOUT THE AUTHORS: BRIAN HUTCHISON & RICHARD GLAZIER

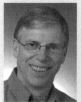

Brian Hutchison is a professor emeritus at McMaster University.

In this month's *Health Affairs*, Brian Hutchison and Richard Glazier offer an analysis of recent reforms in primary care in Ontario, Canada's most populous province. The reforms, designed to improve access to care, patient and provider satisfaction, care quality, and health system efficiency and sustainability, included patient enrollment with a primary care provider; funding for interprofessional primary care organizations; and physician reimbursement arrangements based on varying blends of fee-for-service, capitation, and pay-for-performance. With nearly 75 percent of Ontario's population now enrolled in these new models, the authors highlight some early results and ongoing challenges. In particular, they emphasize the need for ongoing investment in the new models despite fiscal constraints and for a clearly

articulated policy road map to continue the transformation.

Hutchison is a professor emeritus in the Department of Family Medicine and the Department of Clinical Epidemiology and Biostatistics at McMaster University, cochair of the Canadian Working Group for Primary Healthcare Improvement, and senior adviser for primary care to Health Quality Ontario. His areas of research and policy interest include the organization, funding, and delivery of primary and community care; needs-based health care resource allocation and funding methods; provider payment methods; quality improvement; and preventive care. He has a master's degree in health research methodology from McMaster University and a medical degree from the University of Western Ontario.

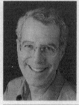

Richard Glazier is a senior scientist at the Institute for Clinical Evaluative Sciences.

Glazier is a senior scientist and program lead of primary care and population health at the Institute for Clinical Evaluative Sciences, in Toronto. He is also a family physician at St. Michael's Hospital, a scientist in the hospital's Centre for Research on Inner City Health, and a professor in the Department of Family and Community Medicine and in the Dalla Lana School of Public Health at the University of Toronto. In addition, he is president-elect of the North American Primary Care Research Group.

Glazier's research focuses on primary care health services delivery models, chronic disease management, health of disadvantaged populations, and equity in health. He received a master's degree in public health from the Johns Hopkins University and a medical degree from the University of Western Ontario.

Attribution

Hutchison B, Glazier R. Ontario's primary care reforms have transformed the local care landscape, but a plan is needed for ongoing improvement. *Health Affairs* 2013;32. doi: 10.1377/hlthaff.2012.1087. Reproduced with permission.

CHAPTER 11

North America: US

Katherine Neuhausen, Kevin Grumbach, Andrew Bazemore and Robert L. Phillips

COORDINATION & INTEGRATION

DOI: 10.1377/hlthaff.2011.1261
HEALTH AFFAIRS 31,
NO. 8 (2012): 1708–1716
©2012 Project HOPE—
The People-to-People Health
Foundation, Inc.

By Katherine Neuhausen, Kevin Grumbach, Andrew Bazemore, and Robert L. Phillips

Integrating Community Health Centers Into Organized Delivery Systems Can Improve Access To Subspecialty Care

Katherine Neuhausen
(kneuhausen@mednet.ucla.edu)
is a Robert Wood Johnson
Foundation Clinical Scholar in
the David Geffen School of
Medicine at the University of
California, Los Angeles.

Kevin Grumbach is chair of
and a professor in the
Department of Family and
Community Medicine at the
University of California, San
Francisco (UCSF), and
codirector of both the UCSF
Center for Excellence in
Primary Care and the UCSF
Clinical and Translational
Science Institute's Community
Engagement and Health Policy
Program.

Andrew Bazemore is medical
director of policy research at
the Robert Graham Center for
Policy Studies in Primary
Care, in Washington, D.C.

Robert L. Phillips is director
of the Robert Graham Center
for Policy Studies in Primary
Care.

ABSTRACT The Affordable Care Act is funding the expansion of
community health centers to increase access to primary care, but this
approach will not ensure effective access to subspecialty services. To
address this issue, we interviewed directors of twenty community health
centers. Our analysis of their responses led us to identify six unique
models of how community health centers access subspecialty care, which
we called Tin Cup, Hospital Partnership, Buy Your Own Subspecialists,
Telehealth, Teaching Community, and Integrated System. We determined
that the Integrated System model appears to provide the most
comprehensive and cohesive access to subspecialty care. Because Medicaid
accountable care organizations encourage integrated delivery of care, they
offer a promising policy solution to improve the integration of
community health centers into "medical neighborhoods."

Community health centers are the
cornerstones of medical care for
many underserved communities
and currently deliver care to nearly
twenty million people.[1] Serving a
patient population of which 37.5 percent is uninsured and 38.5 percent is on Medicaid, community health centers are critical to the primary
care safety net.[2] Over the past decade, the federal
government invested heavily in the expansion of
community health centers.[3] The Affordable Care
Act provides an additional $11 billion to commu-
nity health centers from 2011 to 2015 to help
them meet the rise in demand for primary care
created by the law's broadening of health insurance coverage. However, recent federal budget
cuts may limit the growth of community health
centers.[4]

This expansion of the number and capacity of
community health centers presents major opportunities and challenges for community
health centers. The centers' expansion has focused on increasing access to primary care medical homes.[5] However, although necessary, medi-

cal homes are not sufficient to provide high-
quality health care. In addition to primary care,
patients require a "medical neighborhood"—a
full constellation of coordinated services, including subspecialty and diagnostic services—to
meet their comprehensive health care needs.[6]

Community health centers face substantial
problems in ensuring that their patients receive
subspecialty care.[7,8] A Commonwealth Fund survey found that 91 percent of community health
centers reported difficulty obtaining off-site subspecialty care for uninsured patients.[9] Access
was only slightly easier for patients enrolled in
state and federal insurance programs; 71 percent
of community health centers had difficulty connecting Medicaid patients with subspecialty
care, and 49 percent had trouble obtaining subspecialty care for Medicare patients.[9]

These difficulties affect many patients because
approximately 25 percent of visits to community
health centers require referrals for subspecialty
care and diagnostic services not available at the
center.[10] The challenge of obtaining subspecialty
care in these settings will become even greater in

2014, when millions of Americans newly eligible for Medicaid are expected to seek care at community health centers.[4]

Just such an increase in demand for community health centers was observed after the expansion of insurance coverage in Massachusetts.[11] As community health centers across the nation see more patients, the need for access to subspecialty care is likely to increase, too.

Although studies[9,10] have documented the challenges that community health centers face in accessing subspecialty care for their patients, little is known about how they succeed in doing so. We conducted a study to explore how community health centers arrange access to subspecialty care and build medical neighborhoods that support their medical homes.

Study Data And Methods

DATA COLLECTION We conducted semistructured interviews with the executive director or medical director at twenty community health centers in sixteen states and the District of Columbia from September to October 2010. First, directors representing six community health centers who participated in a data tool training session were invited to participate in the study. These initial interviews were conducted in person at the National Association of Community Health Centers Community Health Institute, in Dallas, Texas.

To identify subjects for the second stage of interviews, we used snowball sampling, in which our initial six subjects recommended some of their colleagues. Staff members at the National Association of Community Health Centers also helped identify centers with innovative models of obtaining subspecialty care.

Based on these recommendations, we contacted an additional twenty-five community health centers by e-mail. Fourteen of these centers agreed to participate and identified their medical director or executive director. These fourteen subjects were interviewed by phone.

The interviews included open-ended questions about how the community health centers accessed subspecialty care for their patients (see Appendix Exhibit 1 for a list of questions).[12] Each participant was asked to rank his or her level of satisfaction with the center's ability to obtain subspecialty care for patients. We used a five-point Likert scale to quantify the respondent's subjective level of satisfaction, from very dissatisfied to very satisfied.

ANALYSIS We discontinued the interviews when saturation was reached for identified themes. After twenty interviews, we decided that additional interviews would not provide any further insight into how community health centers access subspecialty care.

To generate new theory, we used a modified grounded theory method, which is an approach for looking systematically at qualitative data of the sort we had collected in our interview transcripts. Two researchers generated consensus codes for each model by identifying codes that they mutually agreed on. An iterative process was used that allowed new models and themes to arise inductively from the data.

The consensus codes were triangulated among three of the authors to reach consensus on final models and themes. In rare cases of disagreement regarding models or themes, the fourth author was invited to reconcile such disagreements.

The study was approved by the University of California, San Francisco, Committee on Human Research.

LIMITATIONS Our study had several limitations. Because it relied on qualitative interviews with a snowball sample of health center directors, it was exploratory and not necessarily representative of all community health centers. We attempted to capture potential regional and geographic differences by including community health centers from diverse regions and representing a balance of urban and rural settings. Still, our findings are likely to be most valid for community health centers that are similar to the centers that participated in our study.

We also attempted to include the most innovative models by asking the National Association of Community Health Centers, the national professional association for community health centers, to recommend community health centers that they recognized as leaders in implementing innovative models of specialty care access. Therefore, the twenty centers in our study may not represent the full range of models of subspecialty care access.

This is not meant to be an exhaustive or generalizable study of how all community health centers obtain subspecialty care for their patients. Rather, it is a starting point for creating a typology of the models employed by community health centers. It should also help inform policy considerations in this area.

Study Results

The community health centers in our study varied greatly in size, with the number of service sites ranging from two to forty-six. The mean number of sites per health center was 17.5 (Exhibit 1). The number of patients annually receiving care at the community health centers ranged from just under 3,000 to more than 113,000. The mean number of patients was more

EXHIBIT 1

Characteristics Of Twenty Community Health Centers In The Subspecialty Care Access Study, 2010

Characteristic	Mean number/percent
Service delivery sites[a]	17.5
Unduplicated patients served in 2009	45,724
MEAN PATIENT RACE/ETHNICITY[b]	
American Indian	1.5%
Asian	3.3
Black	15.5
Hispanic/Latino[c]	35.5
More than one race	1.1
Pacific Islander	2.2
Unreported/refused to answer	11.8
White	29.0
MEAN PATIENT INSURANCE CHARACTERISTICS	
Medicaid	42.7%
Medicare	6.9
Private insurance	13.7
Other public insurance (non-CHIP)	5.5
Other public insurance (CHIP)	1.6
Uninsured	29.6
LOCATION	
Rural	40.0%
Urban	60.0
GEOGRAPHIC REGION	
Midwest	10.0%
Northeast	35.0
South/southeast	15.0
West	40.0
SERVICES AVAILABLE ON SITE	
Behavioral health	90.0%
Diagnostic laboratory	65.0
Diagnostic radiology	50.0
Oral health	95.0
Pharmacy	65.0

SOURCE Analysis by the Robert Graham Center for Policy Studies in Family Medicine and Primary Care of service area data from the Health Resources and Services Administration Bureau of Primary Health Care Uniform Data System, 2009. **NOTE** CHIP is the Children's Health Insurance Program. [a]Service delivery sites include dental and school-based clinics as well as primary care clinics. [b]Averages for patient racial characteristics are reported by each health center to the Health Resources and Services Administration. [c]Patients who reported Hispanic/Latino ethnicity were counted in the Hispanic/Latino category regardless of whether they also specified a race (such as white or black), to avoid double counting.

than 45,000. On average, 42.7 percent of each center's patients were Medicaid beneficiaries and 29.6 percent were uninsured. Many of the centers provided on-site services.

Obtaining Subspecialty Care: Six Models

We identified six unique models of how the community health centers in our study obtained subspecialty care. We developed our models based on how the centers dealt with referrals to adult medical and surgical subspecialists because these were the most common referrals discussed in our interviews.

MODEL 1: TIN CUP This model, in which health center providers rely on personal relationships to solicit care from an informal network of subspecialists, was the most prevalent one.[13] The community health centers depend on the goodwill of subspecialists to provide charity care to uninsured patients. We refer to this as the Tin Cup model because the solicitations that take place can be viewed as a form of begging.

The El Rio Community Health Center in Tucson, Arizona, increased the Tin Cup model's viability by ensuring that referrals of uninsured patients were evenly distributed.[14] Each month, El Rio sent all physicians in its referral network reports that summarized how many patients were seen by each subspecialist. By presenting evidence that everyone in the community of subspecialists was contributing equally, El Rio strengthened the altruism on which the Tin Cup model depends.

MODEL 2: HOSPITAL PARTNERSHIP In this model, the community health center negotiates a contract with a community hospital to provide subspecialty care. Community health centers affiliated with hospitals usually have better access to subspecialty care than those without hospital affiliations.[9,10] However, many community hospitals have limited numbers of subspecialists on staff. As a result, community health centers must stitch together a patchwork referral system combining hospital-based subspecialty care with other community-based subspecialists.

Building formal partnerships with community hospitals creates opportunities for innovation. At the time of our study, Thundermist Health Center in Rhode Island was introducing a health information exchange with three community hospitals in order to allow interoperability among their electronic health record systems.[14] Hospital affiliations would enable Thundermist to implement its new system across a full spectrum of hospital-based subspecialists.

MODEL 3: BUY YOUR OWN SUBSPECIALISTS In this model, the health center hires its own subspecialists to provide care at a designated specialty hub. Community health centers typically pay subspecialists an hourly rate and receive higher cost-based Medicaid and Medicare prospective payment rates for subspecialty care delivered on site. However, procedurally oriented subspecialists working in community health centers may not have the necessary facilities, equipment, and support staff to perform procedures.

One of the community health centers implementing this model, Unity Health Care in Washington, D.C., had an extensive cadre of employed subspecialists.[14] Unity's thirteen sites referred patients to a multispecialty hub. Unity had two financial advantages: contracts with two Medicaid managed care organizations and a partnership with the DC HealthCare Alliance, a District of Columbia program that paid for primary and subspecialty care for uninsured residents. These funding streams covered the full spectrum of care for Medicaid and uninsured patients and allowed Unity to hire a variety of subspecialists.

MODEL 4: TELEHEALTH This model uses telecommunications equipment to create real-time interactive communication between patients and subspecialists. At the time of our study, Open Door Community Health Center was pioneering the use of telemedicine in rural northern California.[15] Open Door paid subspecialists an hourly rate to work one or two sessions per week at its Telehealth and Visiting Specialist Center. The subspecialists provided telemedicine consultations to patients at Open Door's seven primary care sites. Most of these subspecialists also committed to providing indicated procedures in other settings if those procedures could not be performed at the health center.

Urban safety-net programs have also been adopting novel telehealth strategies. The innovative "eReferral" system developed by San Francisco General Hospital and community clinics enables two-way electronic communication between primary care providers and subspecialists. The program has significantly decreased wait times for subspecialty consultations.[16]

MODEL 5: TEACHING COMMUNITY This model features teaching community health centers that train primary care resident physicians.[17] These centers rely on the collaborative dynamic created when subspecialists are integrated into a health center as teaching faculty.

At the time of our study, the Family Health Center of Worcester, Massachusetts, attributed its strong referral network to its role as a teaching health center that trained University of Massachusetts family medicine residents.[18] Volunteer subspecialists offered podiatry, obstetrics or gynecology, and otolaryngology services at the health center.

The Family Health Center referred patients to subspecialists at the University of Massachusetts Memorial Medical Center, where residents had inpatient rotations. The Family Health Center's teaching connection with the hospital strengthened the relationships that are integral to obtaining subspecialty care.

MODEL 6: INTEGRATED SYSTEM This model features community health centers that are completely integrated with a local government health system or a safety-net hospital that has a comprehensive network of subspecialists.

One of the organizations implementing this model, Denver Health, in Colorado, has been called a model integrated system.[19] Denver Health's network of community health centers (called Denver Community Health Services) included eight federally funded community health centers that delivered primary care under an umbrella of organizations governed by the Denver Health and Hospital Authority. The community health centers were integrated with the Denver Health public hospital, and the centers' patients had access to all subspecialists at the hospital. The centers and the hospital shared a single electronic health record system and web-based referral platform.

Satisfaction With Subspecialty Access

Community health centers that used different models had differing perceptions of ease of access to subspecialty care, with the Tin Cup and Integrated System models at opposite ends of the spectrum. The eight community health centers in this study that used the Tin Cup model struggled the most, with four reporting that they were dissatisfied and three reporting they were neutral regarding their ability to access subspecialty care. All three community health centers using the Integrated System model were very satisfied with their ability to access subspecialty care for their patients.

The other four models fell between the Tin Cup and Integrated System models on the five-point scale. The Hospital Partnership and Buy Your Own Specialist models were employed by three community health centers each, and in each set of three, only one health center was satisfied with its access to subspecialty care using that model. The one health center using the Telehealth model was satisfied with its subspecialty care access. Of the two community health centers using the Teaching Community model, one was neutral and the other was very satisfied.

Discussion

Although the Tin Cup model has been previously described, our study identified five other unique models that community health centers use to arrange subspecialty care. Fitzhugh Mullan has characterized the Tin Cup model as the "perpetual, frustrating, quixotic, creative, and demeaning process of begging for services from others for our patients."[20] More community health centers in our study used this inferior model of obtaining subspecialty care than any other model.

The Integrated System model appears to be the most successful approach to constructing a well-functioning medical neighborhood for community health centers. All three community health centers using this model gave access to subspecialty care the highest rating—a far better evaluation than any other model.

Beyond access to care, directors of community health centers using the Integrated System model reported improved communication, increased coordination of care, and seamless care transitions. Shared electronic health records enabled primary care providers to communicate clearly with subspecialists and avoid duplication of diagnostic testing. Patients were rarely lost to follow-up and experienced improved care transitions between the health center and the hospital.

Our findings suggest that community health centers using any of the other models should transition to the Integrated System model, wherever possible. This model may not be attainable for every health center, however, given the facilitators and barriers present in their communities (see Appendix Exhibit 2 for the key elements, facilitators, and barriers for each model).[12] Community health centers that are not ready to develop or to become part of an integrated system could investigate the other models that exist along the continuum between the fragmented Tin Cup model and the comprehensive Integrated System model.

Policy Implications

Policy makers should use payment reform to support community health center initiatives to move toward or become a part of integrated systems. Investments in integrated systems have the potential to generate considerable returns for federal and state governments, because community health centers will have to absorb much of the increased demand for care as a result of Medicaid expansion under health care reform.

Accountable care organizations hold great potential as instruments for promoting a more integrated model of subspecialty care for community health centers. The Centers for Medicare and Medicaid Services has launched several different types of Medicare accountable care organization initiatives and will allow community health centers to lead Medicare accountable care organizations.[21] However, community health centers have a greater incentive to participate in Medicaid accountable care organizations than Medicare accountable care organizations because 38.5 percent of the centers' patients are enrolled in Medicaid, whereas only 7.5 percent are Medicare beneficiaries.[2]

In the absence of any federal Medicaid accountable care organization initiatives to date, various states are moving forward with legislation to support Medicaid accountable care organizations. Community health centers are participating in a Medicaid accountable care organization in Camden, New Jersey, supported by state legislation.[22] Community health centers in Chicago are equal partners in an innovative Medicaid pilot project called the Medical Home Network,[23] and two different integrated care initiatives in Los Angeles are positioned to become Medicaid accountable care organizations.[24]

Because Medicaid is a federal-state partnership, federal policy must be clearly articulated so that states can develop the shared savings payment model integral to Medicaid accountable care organizations. The Center for Medicare and Medicaid Innovation should support promising state and community accountable care organization initiatives by developing a Medicaid accountable care organization pilot program.

The Medicaid accountable care organization, offering as it does the possibility of shared savings, is a promising financial model for supporting health center initiatives to achieve integrated delivery systems. Shared savings could reward community health centers for the downstream savings from decreased hospitalizations and emergency department visits. However, the accountable care organization model will need to be adapted if the community health centers that are leading Medicaid accountable care organizations are to overcome barriers. Obstacles such as scarce access to start-up seed capital, inadequate infrastructure, limited financial reserves, slow payment cycles, and lack of experience with taking on financial risk may prevent centers from launching such organizations because they are concerned about their financial viability.

First, the Center for Medicare and Medicaid Innovation should provide seed capital funding and technical advisers to help community health centers build the infrastructure for Medicaid accountable care organizations. This support is essential because most centers do not have adequate chronic care management, information technology, or the related infrastructure required for well-functioning accountable care organizations.

Second, the Centers for Medicare and Medicaid Services and state Medicaid agencies should share savings on a first-dollar basis with community health centers, take a lower percentage of the shared savings in the first few years, and offer a five-year initial contract to Medicaid accountable care organizations. Because Medicaid patients on average use fewer health care services than Medicare patients, Medicaid accountable care organizations will realize a smaller amount of shared savings over a longer time period. To achieve meaningful savings, Medicaid accountable care organizations should implement intensive care-management and care-transition programs that target the highest-cost Medicaid patients. Improved care coordination could decrease costs for these patients by reducing preventable emergency department visits and hospitalizations.

Third, Medicaid accountable care organizations should cover the entire population of Medicaid patients in a defined geographical area. This will require the Medicaid accountable care organization to include all of the safety-net hospitals as well as a critical mass of community health centers in that area. Basing patient assignment on geographical location recognizes that many vulnerable patients move between several different safety-net providers in a community.

Fourth, the Innovation Center should consider a special track for teaching community health centers that partner with academic medical centers. Richard Rieselbach and Arthur Kellermann proposed a different model, called Community Health Center and Academic Medical Partnerships, that would enable teaching community health centers to access subspecialists at academic medical centers while anchoring the accountable care organizations in the teaching community health centers' comprehensive approach to primary care.[25]

Finally, the Innovation Center should structure Medicaid accountable care organizations so that community health centers and other providers have no downside financial risk for the initial five years, similar to the savings-only track offered to Medicare accountable care organizations. Community health centers are unlikely to consider a dramatically different payment model unless they are protected from financial losses initially. If the centers achieve meaningful savings under a one-sided savings-only model, they could be transitioned to a two-sided financial risk model with shared savings or losses over time. Policy makers may reconsider the cost-based Medicaid and Medicare prospective payment rates to community health centers if the centers are able to increase revenues under these types of risk-sharing models.

Medicaid accountable care organizations can help community health centers overcome the serious financial obstacles to developing integrated delivery systems without incurring much financial risk themselves. The only risk is that of losing the initial investment in chronic care managers or information technology systems if shared savings are not generated. However, the seed capital would cover much of these initial costs. Even if a Medicaid accountable care organization were to generate excess costs over its initial benchmark, the health center would be held harmless under the savings-only model.

Some community health centers have already shown that they can succeed after taking on more extensive risk under capitation models. Unity Health Care, in Washington, D.C., managed risk by being both the service provider and the insurer under its Medicaid managed care contract. Lawndale Christian Health Center, in Chicago, receives capitated payments for all ambulatory services—including primary care, pharmaceutical benefits, subspecialty services, and emergency care—for much of its Medicaid, Medicare, and commercially insured populations (Arthur Jones, former chief executive officer of Lawndale Christian Health Center, personal communication, March 2, 2012). These community health centers have demonstrated that they can handle much greater risk than would be required to lead an accountable care organization.

Although the Integrated System model, which could be supported by Medicaid accountable care organizations, appears to be the most successful approach, it is also the most challenging to build. For community health centers that cannot yet make the leap to integrated systems, policy makers should support the adoption of the Buy Your Own Subspecialist or Telehealth model. The Health Resources and Services Administration should create a fast-track process to approve applications by community health centers to expand their scope of practice to include subspecialty care. Congress should modify Medicaid and Medicare payment policies to create adequate reimbursement for telemedicine visits and to provide sustainable funding for telehealth programs.

Conclusion

The rapid expansion of community health centers under the Affordable Care Act presents major challenges and unique opportunities for the integration of primary and subspecialty care. Increasing the number of community health centers so that more low-income patients can access primary care necessitates a commensurate increase in access to subspecialty care. Only in this way will the full benefit of safety-net services be realized. Full integration of health services has the potential to turn medical homes into successful medical neighborhoods.

We identified six unique models of how community health centers access subspecialty care and assessed the level of satisfaction with these models among health center directors. We determined that the Integrated System model appears to provide the most comprehensive and cohesive

COORDINATION & INTEGRATION

access to subspecialty care. Based on our findings, we proposed policies and related incentives that could promote health systems integration and create medical neighborhoods in the safety net. These policies should be implemented rapidly to prepare community health centers to provide integrated care to the millions of newly insured patients under health care reform. ■

An earlier version of this manuscript was presented at the North American Primary Care Association's Annual Meeting in Banff, Alberta, on November 15, 2011. The authors are grateful to the medical directors and executive directors who participated in this study. They thank Sean Finnegan for assistance with data analysis. They also thank Tom Bodenheimer, Kara Odom Walker, and Erin Karnes for their thoughtful comments on earlier drafts. The information and opinions contained in research from the Robert Graham Center do not necessarily reflect the views or policy of the American Academy of Family Physicians.

NOTES

1 Adashi EY, Geiger HJ, Fine MD. Health care reform and primary care—the growing importance of the community health center. N Engl J Med. 2010;362(22):2047–50.

2 Health Resources and Services Administration. Selected patient characteristics: 2010 national data [Internet]. Rockville (MD): HRSA; [cited 2011 Nov 15]. Available from: http://bphc.hrsa.gov/uds/socioeconomic.aspx?year=2010&state=

3 Shin P, Bruen B, Jones E, Ku L, Rosenbaum S. The economic stimulus: gauging the early effects of ARRA funding on health centers and medically underserved populations and communities [Internet]. Washington (DC): George Washington University School of Public Health and Health Services; 2010 Feb 16 [cited 2012 Jul 18]. (Geiger Gibson/RCHN Community Health Foundation Research Collaborative Policy Research Brief No. 17). Available from: http://www.gwumc.edu/sphhs/departments/healthpolicy/dhp_publications/pub_uploads/dhpPublication_C41AE130-5056-9D20-3D65728F2361CFAF.pdf

4 Shin P, Rosenbaum S, Paradise J. Community health centers: the challenge of growing to meet the need for primary care in medically underserved communities [Internet]. Washington (DC): Kaiser Commission on Medicaid and the Uninsured; 2012 Mar [cited 2012 Jul 18]. Available from: http://www.kff.org/uninsured/upload/8098-02.pdf

5 Clarke RM, Tseng C, Brook R, Brown AF. Tool used to assess how well community health centers function as medical homes may be flawed. Health Aff (Millwood). 2012;31(3):627–35.

6 Fisher ES. Building a medical neighborhood for the medical home. N Engl J Med. 2008;359(12):1202–5.

7 Felt-Lisk S, McHugh M, Howell E. Monitoring local safety-net providers: do they have adequate capacity? Health Aff (Millwood). 2002;21(5):277–83.

8 Gusmano MK, Fairbrother G, Park H. Exploring the limits of the safety net: community health centers and care for the uninsured. Health Aff (Millwood). 2002;21(6):188–94.

9 Doty MM, Abrams MK, Hernandez SE, Stremikis K, Beal AC. Enhancing the capacity of community health centers to achieve high performance: findings from the 2009 Commonwealth Fund national survey of federally qualified health centers [Internet]. New York (NY): Commonwealth Fund; 2010 May [cited 2011 Nov 15]. Available from: http://www.commonwealthfund.org/~/media/Files/Publications/Fund%20Report/2010/May/1392_Doty_enhancing_capacity_community_hlt_ctrs_2009_FQHC_survey_v4.pdf

10 Cook NL, Hicks LS, O'Malley AJ, Keegan T, Guadagnoli E, Landon BE. Access to specialty care and medical services in community health centers. Health Aff (Millwood). 2007; 26(5):1459–68.

11 Ku L, Jones E, Shin P, Byrne FR, Long SK. Safety-net providers after health care reform: lessons from Massachusetts. Arch Intern Med. 2011;171(15):1379–84.

12 To access the Appendix, click on the Appendix link in the box to the right of the article online.

13 Isaacs SL, Jellinek P. Is there a (volunteer) doctor in the house? Free clinics and volunteer physician referral networks in the United States. Health Aff (Millwood). 2007; 26(3):871–6.

14 The descriptions of the community health centers that use each model are based on the interviews conducted for this study, which included specific questions about how each site operates.

15 California HealthCare Foundation. Chronicling an entry into telehealth: Open Door Community Health Centers [Internet]. Oakland (CA): CHCF; 2010 Apr [cited 2012 Jul 18]. (Issue Brief). Available from: http://www.chcf.org/~/media/MEDIA%20LIBRARY%20Files/PDF/O/PDF%20OpenDoorTelehealth.pdf

16 Chen AH, Kushel MB, Grumbach K, Yee HF. A safety-net system gains efficiencies through "eReferrals" to specialists. Health Aff (Millwood). 2010;29(5):969–71.

17 Morris CG, Johnson B, Kim S, Chen F. Training family physicians in community health centers: a health workforce solution. Fam Med. 2008;40(4):271–6.

18 Knight K, Miller C, Talley R, Yastic M, McColgan K, Proser M, et al. Health centers' contributions to training tomorrow's physicians [Internet]. Washington (DC): National Association of Community Health Centers; 2010 Aug [cited 2012 Jul 18]. Available from: http://www.nachc.com/client/FINAL%20THC%20REPORT%20-%2010222010-1.pdf

19 Gabow P, Eisert S, Wright R. Denver Health: a model for the integration of a public hospital and community health centers. Ann Intern Med. 2003;138(2):143–9.

20 Mullan F. Tin-cup medicine. Health Aff (Millwood). 2001;20(6):217.

21 Centers for Medicare and Medicaid Services. Shared Savings Program [Internet]. Baltimore (MD): CMS; [last modified 2012 May 29; cited 2012 Jul 18]. Available from: http://www.cms.gov/Medicare/Medicare-Fee-for-Service-Payment/sharedsavingsprogram/

22 Brenner J, Highsmith N. An ACO is born in Camden, but can it flourish in Medicaid? Health Affairs Blog [blog on the Internet]. 2011 Jun 23 [cited 2012 Jun 22]. Available from: http://healthaffairs.org/blog/2011/06/23/an-aco-is-born-in-camden-but-can-it-flourish-in-medicaid/

23 Medical Home Network [home page on the Internet]. Chicago (IL): MHN; 2012 [cited 2012 Mar 26]. Available from: http://www.mhnchicago.org

24 National Health Foundation. Integration of emerging healthcare delivery systems in South Los Angeles [Internet]. Los Angeles (CA): NHF; 2011 Jun 7 [cited 2012 Jul 18]. Available from: http://www.nhfca.org/reports/Integration_of_Emerging_Healthcare_Delivery-_S_LA.pdf

25 Rieselbach RE, Kellermann AL. A model health care delivery system for Medicaid. N Engl J Med. 2011; 364(26):2476–8.

ABOUT THE AUTHORS: KATHERINE NEUHAUSEN, KEVIN GRUMBACH, ANDREW BAZEMORE & ROBERT L. PHILLIPS

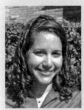

Katherine Neuhausen is a Robert Wood Johnson Foundation Clinical Scholar in the UCLA David Geffen School of Medicine.

providers, and access to primary care for underserved populations. She earned a medical degree from Emory University and completed her family medicine residency training at the University of California, San Francisco (UCSF), and San Francisco General Hospital.

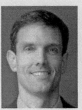

Andrew Bazemore is the medical director of policy research at the Robert Graham Center for Policy Studies in Primary Care.

In this month's *Health Affairs*, Katherine Neuhausen and coauthors report on interviews they conducted with directors of twenty community health centers to determine how they accessed subspecialty care on behalf of patients. The authors identified six different models that these centers pursued and determined that those centers that become an actual or de facto part of an integrated system appeared to provide the most comprehensive and cohesive subspecialty access. The authors suggest that Medicaid accountable care organizations offer a promising policy solution to improve the integration of community health centers into "medical neighborhoods."

Neuhausen is a Robert Wood Johnson Foundation Clinical Scholar in the David Geffen School of Medicine at the University of California, Los Angeles (UCLA). She is a clinical instructor in the UCLA Department of Family Medicine and practices family medicine at the Mid Valley Family Health Center, which is operated by the Los Angeles County Department of Health Services. She is also an investigator for a RAND Corporation study funded by the Commonwealth Fund on developing integrated care systems for low-income populations.

Neuhausen's research interests include the financing of safety-net health systems, new payment models that support delivery system reform for Medicaid

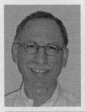

Kevin Grumbach is chair of and a professor in the Department of Family and Community Medicine, UCSF.

Kevin Grumbach is chair of and a professor in the Department of Family and Community Medicine at UCSF, codirector of the UCSF Center for Excellence in Primary Care, and codirector of the UCSF Clinical and Translational Science Institute's Community Engagement and Health Policy Program. He has extensive experience in conducting health services and clinical and translational research, with an emphasis on primary care, disparities in health care, how to improve health care delivery in the primary care setting, and participatory models of evaluation research, including implementation and dissemination science.

Grumbach is also a member of the *Annals of Family Medicine* editorial board and the Institute of Medicine. In 2012 he was awarded the UCSF Chancellor's Public Service Award and the Society of Teachers of Family Medicine's Advocacy Award. He received a medical degree from UCSF and completed his residency training in family medicine at San Francisco General Hospital.

Andrew Bazemore is the medical director of policy research at the Robert Graham Center for Policy Studies in Primary Care. The center's goal is to improve individual and population health by enhancing the delivery of primary care. Bazemore directs research and projects related to access to care for underserved populations, the health workforce, spatial analysis and health, and other topics. He is an associate professor in the University of Cincinnati's Department of Family Medicine and serves on the faculty of the Department of Family Medicine at Georgetown University and in the Department of Health Policy at the George Washington University School of Public Health.

Bazemore earned a medical degree from the University of North Carolina and a master's degree in public health from Harvard University. He was chief resident of international health in the University of Cincinnati's Family Practice Residency Program.

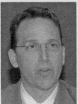

Robert L. Phillips is director of the Robert Graham Center for Policy Studies in Primary Care.

Robert Phillips is director of the Robert Graham Center for Policy Studies in Primary Care. He is

COORDINATION & INTEGRATION

currently principal investigator on a study of graduate medical education accountability measures that will inform issues of stewardship related to $13 billion spent on these programs annually. Phillips also serves on a number of boards. He is a board member of the North American Primary Care Research Group and a member of the Institute of Medicine's Integration of Public Health and Primary Care Study Committee.

Phillips is a member of the Institute of Medicine and a Fulbright Specialist, serving at the request of other countries to advise on various primary care research topics. He earned a medical degree from the University of Florida and a master's degree in public health from the University of Missouri.

Attribution

Neuhausen K, Grumbach K, Bazemore A, Phillips RL. Integrating community health centers into organized delivery systems can improve access to subspecialty care. *Health Affairs* 2012;31:1708–1716. doi: 10.1377/hlthaff.2011.1261. Reproduced with permission.

CHAPTER 12

North America: Mexico

Chris van Weel, Deborah Turnbull, José Ramirez, Andrew Bazemore, Richard H. Glazier, Carlos Jaen, Bob Phillips and Jon Salsberg

SUPPORTING HEALTH REFORM IN MEXICO: EXPERIENCES AND SUGGESTIONS FROM AN INTERNATIONAL PRIMARY HEALTH CARE CONFERENCE

Primary care is essential for sustainable health care.[1] Mexico is undergoing socioeconomic and health care developments, but a barrier is policy makers' poor understanding of the role and function of primary care. Consequently, the country struggles to meet the health needs of its population. The Mexican College of Family Medicine (MCFM) has the potential to lead health systems change with strong primary care, but lacks capacity. A pre-conference at the 2015 Cancun NAPCRG conference aimed to develop an action plan and build leadership capacity for MCFM (http://www.napcrg.org/Resources/CancunManifesto/SupportingHealthReforminMexico-FullPaper).

International Collaboration

There is substantial international experience in implementing primary care policy to reform health systems.[2-7] This policy implementation requires translating general principles of primary care to local circumstances and priorities; articulating primary care's contribution to population health (ie advocacy); and engaging with multiple stakeholders in a bottom-up process to address population needs.

Mexican Health (Care)

Mexico is experiencing a demographic transition, with an aging population and an increase in chronic diseases (notably diabetes mellitus).[8]

Since 1943 the Mexican Health System has covered various sectors of the population. Additional legislation was introduced in 2014[9,10] and upgraded in 2015, to ensure full health care coverage.

Despite a convergence of services,[11] each health structure that passed legislation has a vertical financing system which increases administrative expenses. In 2011 these administrative costs represented an estimated 10.8% of total expenditure on health.[9]

Coherent primary care is absent. Primary care is provided, depending on the funder, by institution-certified family physicians, general practitioners, or non-certified family physicians or social service interns.[12] Practice visits are short (12 minutes) and curative in focus, with less than 10% being preventive in nature.[13] Accordingly, family medicine accounts for only 4% of over 26,000 training positions.[14] This gives urgency to focus health reforms on primary care, including financing and training.

In summary, the most urgent issues are:
- Lack of structure and coordination between primary care and hospitals
- Insufficient coverage and access for the many poor
- Insufficient understanding of the primary care role
- Lack of teaching, training, or research of health problems in the community
- Poor socioeconomic status of family physicians

Two International Examples of Success

Ontario, Canada provides a lesson on system transformation through physician payment and interprofessional teams.[15-17] Capitation payment blended with fee-for-service and pay-for-performance incentives became the preferred reimbursement, and about one-quarter of physicians were supported with interprofessional teams.

The health transformation increased physician reimbursement and satisfaction. Students' interest in family medicine almost doubled to 40% of graduates. Important lessons learned were to adjust capitation to populations' health needs and to align primary care incentives with the needs of the rest of the health system.

The US experience, often copied in Central American countries, demonstrates that health investment does not lead to a return in health outcomes,[18] without investment in the primary care function. Additionally, markets with fee-for-service payments create mal-distribution of workforce away from areas with high health needs.

As an alternative, decentralized, local "communities of solution" are powerful in achieving more with less resources, as exemplified in the *Hombro a Hombro project* in Honduras.[19] Through an academic/community partnership, "committees" for health identified social determinants of health needing greatest attention and prioritized resources accordingly.

Learning points for Mexico were:
- Blended capitation payment for primary care
- Describing the main health problems in the population
- Family practice specialty training in the community setting
- Insight into numbers and geographic distribution of health care professionals

Working With Stakeholders

Engagement between care providers, patients and their caregivers, managers, and policy makers improves responses to complex needs.[20-23] To secure patient-centered care, primary care providers and researchers need to engage with those who will ultimately benefit.[24-26] Meaningful engagement results in more rapid uptake of evidence into practice, and more satisfaction with care provided.[27-29]

Problems of working with patients in the Mexican situation were:

• Unavailability of consumer organizations
• Patients passive toward health care professionals
• Patients poorly understood the role of primary care

Conclusion

The meeting participants proposed the *Cancun Manifesto*, an action plan for MCFM to lead a long-term strategy for health reform in Mexico.[30] To increase understanding among stakeholders of the values of primary care, and to advocate its development, short-term objectives were identified:

• Describing the *Mexican* Ecology of Medical Care[31]
• Collecting patients' experiences with their family physician
• Defining role and function of primary care [32] in the Mexican context

International support to the MCFM will continue. This pre-conference process can be used with other countries facing health systems change.

Chris van Weel, Radboud University Nijmegen, The Netherlands, Australian National University, Canberra, Australia; Deborah Turnbull, University of Adelaide, Australia; José Ramirez, Autonomous University of Nuevo Leon in Monterrey NL, Mexico, Mexican Family Physician College; Andrew Bazemore, Robert Graham Center for Policy Studies in Family Medicine & Primary Care, Washington DC; Richard H. Glazier, Institute for Clinical Evaluative Sciences, St. Michaels Hospital, University of Toronto, Canada; Carlos Jaen, The University of Texas Health Science Center at San Antonio, San Antonio, Texas; Bob Phillips, American Board of Family Medicine, Washington, DC, Jon Salsberg, McGill University, Montreal, Canada

References available in pre-conference report at http://www.napcrg.org/Resources/CancunManifesto/SupportingHealthReforminMexico-FullPaper.

Attribution

Weel C van, Turnbull D, Ramirez J, Bazemore A, Glazier RH, Jaen C, Phillips BL, Salsberg J. Supporting health reform in Mexico: Experiences and suggestions from an international primary health care conference. *Annals of Family Medicine* 2016;14:279–280. doi: 10.1370/afm.1942. Reproduced with permission.

CHAPTER 13

South Asia

*Chris van Weel, Ryuki Kassai, Waris Qidwai,
Raman Kumar, Kanu Bala, Pramendra
Prasad Gupta, Ruvaiz Haniffa, Neelamani
Rajapaksa Hewageegana, Thusara Ranasinghe,
Michael Kidd and Amanda Howe*

Analysis

BMJ Global Health

Primary healthcare policy implementation in South Asia

Chris van Weel,[1,2] Ryuki Kassai,[3] Waris Qidwai,[4] Raman Kumar,[5] Kanu Bala,[6] Pramendra Prasad Gupta,[7] Ruvaiz Haniffa,[8] Neelamani Rajapaksa Hewageegana,[9] Thusara Ranasinghe,[10] Michael Kidd,[11] Amanda Howe[12]

To cite: van Weel C, Kassai R, Qidwai W, et al. Primary healthcare policy implementation in South Asia. BMJ Global Health 2016;1:e000057. doi:10.1136/bmjgh-2016-000057

Received 4 April 2016
Revised 23 May 2016
Accepted 25 May 2016

ABSTRACT

Primary healthcare is considered an essential feature of health systems to secure population health and contain costs of healthcare while universal health coverage forms a key to secure access to care. This paper is based on a workshop at the 2016 World Organization of Family Doctors (WONCA) South Asia regional conference, where the health systems of Bangladesh, India, Nepal, Pakistan and Sri Lanka were presented in relation to their provision of primary healthcare. The five countries have in recent years improved the health of their populations, but currently face the challenges of non-communicable diseases and ageing populations. Primary healthcare should be a core component in restructuring health systems. However, there is a lack of understanding among policymakers of the unique contribution of primary healthcare to the health of populations. This results in insufficient investment in facilities and low priority of specialty training in the community setting. Regional collaboration could strengthen the advocacy for primary healthcare to policymakers and other stakeholders. Priorities were investment in community-based health facilities, and access to healthcare through professionals specialty-trained in the primary healthcare setting. This development fits the strategy of the WHO South East Asian Region to use community-based healthcare in achieving universal health coverage for the Asian populations.

Key questions

What is already known about this topic?

► Primary healthcare is an essential component of cost-effective healthcare. Insight into countries' health systems is important to plan effective ways to strengthen health systems. However, for most countries there is limited insight into the role and position of primary healthcare in their system.

What are the new findings?

► This paper provides field experience from five countries which populate a quarter of the world population. Demographic developments require a strengthening of their primary healthcare. However, low investment, poor planning and a lack of understanding of the unique contribution of primary healthcare for population health impede this development.

Recommendations for policy

► Regional collaboration and advocacy for primary healthcare can support countries in an appropriate investment in community-based health services and specialty training of professionals in the primary healthcare setting, and substantially improve access to healthcare.

CrossMark

For numbered affiliations see end of article.

Correspondence to
Professor Chris van Weel;
chris.vanweel@radboudumc.nl

Most countries experience major challenges to their health systems and the South Asian region is no exception. Factors behind this global trend are increasing health costs, and diminished returns on investment for ageing populations. Where the primary healthcare function is formally structured in the health system, and professionals are educated for their specific tasks, the performance of the system is often optimised: better primary healthcare leads to better population health at lower healthcare costs.[1] Strengthening primary healthcare for sustainable healthcare is a global strategy[2] that can benefit from international collaboration.[3] A critical feature of this strategy is the adaptation of general principles to the prevailing local conditions: primary healthcare has to be built-up from the community level where it has to operate.[4] For this a good understanding of the existing health system is important in initiating reforms. There is growing insight in primary healthcare in Europe and North America,[3 5] but for many countries or regions data are scarce.[4] In response to this, the World Organization of Family Doctors (WONCA) took the initiative to document how primary care is organised around the world, and to create dialogues of how the values of primary healthcare are addressed within different health systems.[6 7] A workshop at the 2016 WONCA South Asia regional conference in Colombo, Sri Lanka, offered an opportunity to compare the health systems of five WONCA member countries: Bangladesh, India, Nepal, Pakistan and Sri Lanka.

Universal health coverage (UHC) is a key to secure access to care. The WHO South East Asian Region has promoted a regional UHC strategy centred on community-based healthcare, with family physicians at its core.[8] Services should integrate health promotion, disease prevention, diagnosis, treatment, disease management, rehabilitation and palliative care. Stepwise implementation is designed to adopt the perspectives of individuals, families and communities, in the capacity of participants as well as beneficiaries. Strengthening primary healthcare is considered a cost-effective low risk approach, to make sure that full population coverage is realised ('no one is left behind') by 2030.

This paper is based on the findings of a workshop at the WONCA South Asia conference in Colombo in February 2016, where the field experience of primary healthcare development in five countries—Bangladesh, India, Nepal, Pakistan and Sri Lanka—was presented and discussed with the objective of identifying common strategies for strengthening primary medical healthcare, and priorities for regional collaboration.

Academic family physicians presented a case study of their country, using as a framework a set of 11 power point slides developed by WONCA,[6] each focused on country demographics, the health system and the role and position of primary healthcare, the country's main health challenges, strengths and weakness of the system to address health needs and lessons others could learn from their country. Presenters were free to concentrate on what in their views were the most important information, and subsequently provided a summary of their presentation for this article. Discussion was directed towards regional planning for universal health coverage, how changes towards stronger primary healthcare could occur, and how international collaboration could support this.

These discussions were placed in the context of the regional planning of UHC policy.[8]

SUMMARIES OF COUNTRY CASE STUDIES

Sri Lanka has achieved low maternal and neonatal death rates and high immunisation coverage through the introduction of selective primary healthcare,[9] spending 3.2% of their gross domestic product (GDP). Vertical programmes have been delivered as free primary healthcare by grass root health workers, public health midwifes and public health inspectors. Currently, there is an increased impact of non-communicable and lifestyle-related diseases (NCD) on the health status of the population. To respond to this new challenge, the existing vertical programmes are insufficient: there is the need for a health system that is able to address a range of health problems and integrates health education, prevention and timely intervention directed at the whole person. An important barrier to realise this is that every medical specialist can

practice in the community, without specific professional training for primary healthcare competencies. As a consequence overuse of specialist care and episodic treatment of diseases in isolation stands in the way of continuity of care based on relation of trust over time. This makes the development of strong, comprehensive primary healthcare as the basis of the health system an urgency.

Nepal is a low-and-middle-income country, with significant disparities in health, education, wealth and access to care between Nepal's 126 distinct ethnic/caste groups, and between people living in different regions. The country is making slow but steady progress in improving its population health and well-being, focusing on equity and inclusiveness by health policymakers and professionals spending 1.8% of GDP on health. However, there is a shortage of resources, in particular in rural areas: with only one hospital for every 168 000 persons (a hospital bed for every 4000 rural persons) and a physician for every 92 000 persons (a health post for every 24 000 rural persons). In addition, the limited resources are not used in an optimal way: there is a lack of political commitment for primary healthcare that can respond to all relevant health problems, as the basis of the health system. This results in poor interaction between primary, secondary and tertiary care, and poor integration between government and the private sector with overuse and underuse of resources, and insufficient penetration of health programmes down to the community level, leading to avoidable, low health status of the population.[10 11]

India is the second most populous country in the world. Though the total fertility rate has decreased over the decades, the overall population is steadily increasing. The health sector consists of both private and public providers. The health system is overtly privatised with more than 78% of care provided by the private sector and public investment, at a stable 1% of the total GDP, low.[12] Services are oriented towards tertiary and curative care and due to low insurance coverage care is covered by out of pocket payment. Catastrophic health-related expenditures are leading families into poverty. Services are concentrated in urban areas although 70% of the population live in the rural areas. This is exacerbated by the dual epidemic of NCD—currently accountable for 53% of total deaths—and infectious diseases. In 2005, the Government launched a National Rural Health Mission (NRHM) to strengthen human resources as well as infrastructure focusing on 18 poorly performing states. The NRHM has now evolved into the National Health Mission which also covers the urban health needs.[13] To become truly successful, this mission has to be connected to UHC, but although discussions on UHC gained momentum during the past 5 years with the publication of a strategy for its implementation in 2011[14] this may take some time before it is realised.

Bangladesh is the eighth biggest country of the World with a density of 1033.5/km^2 and with per capita

van Weel C, *et al. BMJ Glob Health* 2016;**1**:e000057. doi:10.1136/bmjgh-2016-000057

BMJ Global Health

income of only $1 314 00. The country is virtually homogeneous in ethnicity, with a landmass of fertile plains and a large delta prone to flooding. On average there is a physician for 3000 people, but this can vary to 1:20 000 and 3.7% of GDP is spent on health.[15] Through vertical public health programmes and other societal interventions the health indicators have substantially improved. However, to achieve UHC and address noncommunicable and lifestyle diseases, there is still a long way to go.

Most inhabitants rely on the private sector and have to pay directly out of their own pockets. Most physicians are 'general practitioners', who have not been professionally trained for primary healthcare competencies. In addition, there is large scale use of complementary and alternative healers. The government has developed a Government Health Delivery System which is inadequate to secure access for all. More recently, through public–private partnerships more than 10 000 community health centres have been established. This has relied substantially on the employment of nurses and hospital trained specialists. It appears the model for the future, but to fully benefit from it specialty training for 'general practitioners' is required as a qualification to work in the primary healthcare setting.

Pakistan is the sixth most populous country in the world and consists largely of young people.[16 17] On paper, the health system is well planned, but a lack of basic human and material resources stand in the way of functioning as designed. On top of this, lack of regulation, renders it non-functional, which results in avoidable, poor health status of the population. The private sector is the main provider of care, with about 80% of healthcare-related expense.[18]

NCD are rising, and related to lifestyle (tobacco smoking in 23% of males, elevated blood pressure in 25% and obesity 5.5% of the population and increasing alcohol consumption and physical inactivity): close to 2000 Pakistanis losing their lives to a preventable noncommunicable disease every day and the probability of dying between ages 30 and 70 years from a NCDs is 21%.[19 20] The Department of Health has responded through vertical NCD units, spending 2.8% of GDP on health. However, an overall lack of operational strategy, including the absence of evidence-based guidelines for its management hamper an effective approach through primary care. Owing to the low priority and limited resources primary healthcare is generally poorly developed, although there have been some excellent models developed through academic outreach.

The presented case studies focused at each country's specific situation. India, with its massive population, devolved state-based health systems, large private health sector and predominantly 'out of pocket' payment, presents a different challenge in securing effective primary healthcare than, for example, Sri Lanka with its historic countrywide approach to public health and population interventions that are free at point of use. These differences will shape their developments in the coming years. However, at the same time, a number of common themes came forward.

The first is financial: the five countries spend <4% of their GDP on health. More importantly, this modest investment is spent in an ineffective way, with an emphasis on hospital—and specialist provided rather than community-based services. The resulting problems for access and equity are further exacerbated by the often substantial out of pocket payments. This emphasises the importance of a coherent strategy to introduce strong community-based primary care with family medicine under UHC.[8]

Second, there is an urgent need in the region for advocacy of a strong primary healthcare function. The WONCA–WHO partnership will help in approaching governments, provide leadership for regional collaboration and engage with other stakeholders (patients/service users, professionals, policymakers, insurers and community leaders) for health system change. A priority is to address the isolated position of primary healthcare and general practice.

Advocacy of health insurance and UHC should include funding conditions that are likely to ensure comprehensive primary healthcare with minimal access barriers for the poor and cover preventive and chronic disease management. There is a tendency to approach UHC without a view on primary healthcare policy.[21 22] This may undermine its realisation, as primary healthcare makes health systems more robust[23] and results in greater equity and more cost-effective care.[1 2] This makes the South East Asian WHO Strategy to combine UHC and primary health a powerful and timely one.[8] It underlines the need of better markers of the complex and integrated contribution primary healthcare makes to population health.[24] Part of this complexity is its contribution to other sectors than healthcare (and healthcare related costs), in pursuing health.[25]

The third point is the establishment of specialty training of general practitioners and other primary healthcare professionals in the primary healthcare setting, by primary healthcare professionals, as the accreditation for patient care in the community. Partnership with universities and regional collaboration through fellowships can help in building capacity and expertise, as has been demonstrated in the Primafamed project in Sub-Saharan Africa.[26]

Among the stakeholders, engagement with patients is of particular importance. One of the problems is that often there are no patient organisations available to recruit from. An alternative, or initial step in helping patients to organise their voice, could be to collect their experiences with their health problems, their self-care and (primary) healthcare professionals. South Asian patients experiences can at the same time provide important qualitative data for cross-national and scholarly collaboration to inform policy towards care that is accessible, affordable, acceptable and effective.

BMJ Global Health

Although the challenges identified from these comparative case studies follow from the specific South Asia context, there are at the same time substantial similarities with challenges encountered in other parts of the world: the importance of a stronger focus on research, teaching and training in the primary healthcare setting, under the leadership of primary healthcare experts through a primary healthcare academic outreach is universal. And this in turn underlines the importance of collaboration beyond the region and the contribution international experts and expertise have to offer for the challenges that are facing South Asia in implementing primary healthcare policy and pursue UHC.

Author affiliations
[1]Department of Primary and Community Care, Radboud University Medical Center, Nijmegen, The Netherlands
[2]Division of Health Services Research and Policy, Research School of Population Health, Australian National University, Acton, Australian Capital Territory, Australia
[3]Department of Community and Family Medicine, Fukushima Medical University, Fukushima, Japan
[4]Department of Family Medicine Service Line Family Health, Aga Khan University, Karachi, Pakistan
[5]Academy of Family Physicians of India, New Delhi, India
[6]Bangladesh Institute of Family Medicine & Research, University of Science & Technology Chittagong, Hatirpool, Dhaka, Bangladesh
[7]Department of General Practice and Emergency Medicine, B.P. Koirala Institute of Health Sciences, Ghopa, Dharan, Nepal
[8]College of General Practitioners of Sri Lanka, Colombo, Sri Lanka
[9]Ministry of Health, Colombo, Sri Lanka
[10]WHO Country Office, Colombo, Sri Lanka
[11]Faculty of Medicine, Nursing and Health Sciences, Flinders University, Adelaide, South Australia, Australia
[12]Norwich Medical School, University of East Anglia, Norwich, Norfolk, UK

Handling editor Seye Abimbola

Contributors CvW designed the outline of the paper, organised the first draft and made the final version. RK, AH and MK commented on the paper outline, revised the first draft and contributed to the final draft. WQ, RK, KB, PPG, RH and NRH contributed their country profile and contributed to the final draft. TR contributed the WHO South-East Asia perspective and contributed to the final draft.

Competing interests None declared.

Provenance and peer review Not commissioned; externally peer reviewed.

Data sharing statement No additional data are available.

REFERENCES
1. Starfield B. Is primary care essential? *Lancet* 1994;344: 1129–33.
2. World Health Organization. *The World Health Report 2008—Primary Healthcare, now more than ever.* Geneva: WHO, 2008. http://www.who.int/whr/2008/en/ (accessed 28 Jan 2016).
3. *J Am Board Fam Med* 2012;25(Suppl 1). http://www.jabfm.org/content/25/Suppl_1.toc (accessed 28 Jan 2016).
4. van Weel C, Turnbull D, Whitehead E, *et al.* International collaboration in innovating health systems. *Ann Fam Med* 2015;13:86–7.
5. Kringos D. *The strength of Primary Care in Europe* [Thesis]. Utrecht, : University of Utrecht, 2012. http://www.nivel.nl/sites/default/files/bestanden/Proefschrift-Dionne-Kringos-The-strength-of-primary-care.pdf (accessed 28 Jan 2016).
6. WONCA Research Working Party Multi-national Plenary Panel Project. http://www.globalfamilydoctor.com/groups/WorkingParties/Research/plenarypanelprojectresourcedocuments.aspx (accessed 28 Jan 2016).
7. Weel C, van Kassai R, *et al.* Evolving health policy for primary care in the Asia Pacific region. *Br J Gen Pract* 2016;66:e451–3.
8. WHO South East Asia Region. Report of the sixty-eighth session. Resolution SEA/RC68/R6 Community-based health services and their contributions to universal health coverage, 2015. http://apps.who.int/iris/bitstream/10665/204455/3/RC68_Report%20.pdf (accessed 28 Aug 2016).
9. Hewa S. Sri Lanka's approach to Primary Healthcare: a success story in South Asia. *GMJ* 2011;16:24–30.
10. Resource Center for Primary Healthcare (RECPHEC). Essential Healthcare Services (EHCS) in Nepal. 2015. http://www.ridanepal.org/downloaded/EHCS%20briefing%20paper.pdf
11. Ministry of Health and Population Nepal, Partnership for Maternal, Newborn & Child Health, WHO, World Bank and Alliance for Health Policy and Systems Research. *Success factors for women's and children's health: Nepal.* Geneva: World Health Organization, 2014.
12. WHO Country Profile: India. http://www.who.int/countries/ind/en/ (accessed 15 Mar 2016).
13. Government of India. National Health Mission of India. http://nrhm.gov.in/nhm.html (accessed 15 Mar 2016).
14. Planning Commission. *High Level Expert Group Report of Universal Health Coverage in India Report 2011.* http://planningcommission.nic.in/reports/genrep/rep_uhc0812.pdf (accessed 15 Mar 2016).
15. WHO. Country profile Bangladesh. http://www.who.int/countries/bgd/en/ (accessed 11 May 2016).
16. WHO Country profile Pakistan. http://www.who.int/gho/countries/pak.pdf?ua=1 (accessed 1 Mar 2016).
17. http://worldpopulationreview.com/countries/pakistan-population/ Health Systems Profile- Pakistan Regional Health Systems Observatory- EMRO http://www.who.int/countries/pak/en/ (accessed 3 Mar 2016).
18. Nishtar S. The Gateway Paper. Health Systems in Pakistan—a Way Forward. http://heartfile.org/pdf/phpf-GWP.pdf (accessed 3 Mar 2016).
19. WHO. Pakistan. http://www.who.int/nmh/countries/pak_en.pdf?ua=1 (accessed 3 Mar 2016).
20. Wasay M, Zaidi S, Jooma R. Non communicable diseases in Pakistan: burden, challenges and way forward for healthcare authorities. *J Pak Med Assoc* 2014;64:1218–19. http://ecommons.aku.edu/pakistan_fhs_mc_med_med/187 (accessed 4 Mar 2016).
21. Reich MR, Harris J, Ikegami N. *et al.* Moving towards universal health coverage: lessons from 11 country studies. *Lancet* 2016;387:811–16.
22. Schmidt H, Gostin LO, Emanuel EJ. Public health, universal health coverage, and Sustainable Development Goals: can they coexist? *Lancet* 2015;386:928–30.
23. World Health Assembly. Resolution 62.12 Primary healthcare, including health system strengthening. 2009. http://apps.who.int/gb/ebwha/pdf_files/WHA62-REC1/WHA62_REC1-en.pdf (accessed 1 Mar 2016).
24. Kidd MR, Padula Anderson MI, Obazee EM, *et al.* The need for global primary care development indicators. *Lancet* 2015;386:737. http://www.thelancet.com/journals/lancet/article/PIIS0140-6736(15)61532-X/abstract
25. Pettigrew LM, De Maeseneer J, Padula Anderson MI, *et al.* Primary healthcare and the Sustainable Development Goals. *Lancet* 2015;386:2119–21. http://www.thelancet.com/journals/lancet/article/PIIS0140-6736(15)00949-6/fulltext?rss%3Dyes
26. Flinkenflögel M, Essuman A, Chege P, *et al.* Family medicine training in sub-Saharan Africa: South-South cooperation in the Primafamed project as strategy for development. *Fam Pract* 2014;31:427–36.

Primary healthcare policy implementation in South Asia

Chris van Weel, Ryuki Kassai, Waris Qidwai, Raman Kumar, Kanu Bala, Pramendra Prasad Gupta, Ruvaiz Haniffa, Neelamani Rajapaksa Hewageegana, Thusara Ranasinghe, Michael Kidd and Amanda Howe

BMJ Glob Health 2016 1:
doi: 10.1136/bmjgh-2016-000057

Updated information and services can be found at:
http://gh.bmj.com/content/1/2/e000057

These include:

References	This article cites 10 articles, 3 of which you can access for free at: http://gh.bmj.com/content/1/2/e000057#BIBL
Open Access	This is an Open Access article distributed in accordance with the Creative Commons Attribution Non Commercial (CC BY-NC 4.0) license, which permits others to distribute, remix, adapt, build upon this work non-commercially, and license their derivative works on different terms, provided the original work is properly cited and the use is non-commercial. See: http://creativecommons.org/licenses/by-nc/4.0/
Email alerting service	Receive free email alerts when new articles cite this article. Sign up in the box at the top right corner of the online article.

Topic Collections	Articles on similar topics can be found in the following collections Open access (78)

Notes

Attribution

Weel C van, Kassai R, Qidwai W, Kumar R, Bala K, Gupta PP, Haniffa R, Hewageegana NR, Ranasinghe T, Kidd M, Howe A. Primary healthcare policy implementation in South Asia. *BMJ Global Health* 2016;1:e000057. doi: 10.1136/bmjgh-2016-000057. Reproduced with permission.

CHAPTER 14

Conclusions: From regional experiences to policy and implementation

Chris van Weel

The first conclusion from Part III is that with the plenary panel project initiative of the WONCA Working Party on Research [1] it has been possible to generate experiences of primary health care development from all regions of the world. This is a most welcome expansion, but at the same time it should be stressed that it is only the beginning of a process – the start of a journey – that should be continued over the coming years.

From this, three consecutive steps have to be taken. Understanding the specific situation in which primary health care is to be strengthened – the local context in which to work – is a critical starting point. And though the experiences that were presented showed great similarities, each national jurisdiction is at the same time particular, and few if any achievements realised in one place can be 'copy-paste' implemented in primary health care elsewhere. Exploring successes and failures comprises the second step, and the power of international comparisons is in that it deepens the understanding of primary health care and how it relates to a country's own situation. Only when this is accomplished will it be possible to take the third step: transfer to the local context. This came strikingly forward in Chapters 10 and 11 but played a role for every country involved.

Yet, at the same time, a number of common issues came forward. Health policy is often restricted to the public sector, while a substantial part of health care – including primary health care – is provided privately. This tension between public and private was emphasised in Chapters 5, 6, 7, 9 and 13 and should be taken into account in primary health care policy. Chapter 14 will look into this, in the context of Asia.

A common problem that is encountered is the failure to integrate health policy and legislation with investment in (primary) health care. This came forward strikingly in the experiences in Latin America, described in Chapter 9. The Ibero-American region has worked very hard in connecting primary health care development in the field to health policy, with tri-annual *primary health care policy summits*, which could be a model of collaborative action for other regions. Also, most countries of the Ibero-American region have access to health care secured in their legislation and connected to universal health coverage. Yet, the progress on the ground is often disappointing, as practising in the community remains under-invested and undervalued.

This is the recurrent issue in connecting legislation to regulations of the health system and to speciality training and professional development in primary health care. Speciality training – in particular in family medicine – is provided in many countries now, rising professional competencies. Yet, often primary health care professionals are unable to execute their competencies because the regulations of the health system only allow them limited tasks and resources. At the same time, the effects of professional training are limited as other specialists, and/or practitioners without any speciality training, are allowed to practice in the primary health care setting.

This stresses the importance of a strong primary health care infrastructure and leadership to influence policy. Primary health care professionals will have the best understanding of the complexity of primary health care and its implications for health reforms. Chapter 12 presented a detailed case study of how to orchestrate an academic-professional basis from which to operate and collaborate. The European experiences (Chapter 8) of the past decade have capitalized on this, and Chapter 15 presents an exciting exploration of how to build regional strength through South–South collaboration in Africa.

In the past decade, policy makers have been supportive of primary health care, in particular for budgetary considerations. But this 'natural' support may change in the current neo-liberal political climate. Primary health care leaders should therefore continue to explore ways to continue the political dialogue and generate evidence in support of the continued development of primary health care. This is further explored in Chapter 16.

The positive contribution to population health – its contribution to the health of poor and rich alike; resilient communities; healthy workforce – have potential under these conditions. This reinforces the importance of access to health care and the importance of mitigating the financial consequences for individuals. This makes the pursuit of *universal health coverage* [2] an international priority. This amplifies the collaboration with the World Health Organization (WHO) and its regional offices. Chapter 17 explores this further.

REFERENCES

1. WONCA. *WONCA research working party multi-national plenary panel project.* Retrieved from: http://www.globalfamilydoctor.com/site/DefaultSite/filesystem/documents/Groups/Research/WONCA%20Research%20Panel%20project.pdf (accessed 28 Jan 2016).
2. WHO. Universal Health Coverage. Retrieved from: http://www.who.int/universal_health_coverage/en/ (accessed May 1, 2017).

PART IV

FROM DATA TO POLICY

CHAPTER 15

Analysis of findings in Asia

Chris van Weel and Ryuki Kassai

BMJ 2017;356:j634 doi: 10.1136/bmj.j634 (Published 2017 February 27)

Check for updates

ANALYSIS

Expanding primary care in South and East Asia

Chris van Weel and **Ryuki Kassai** look at efforts to strengthen primary care and call for regional and international collaboration to help implement policy

Chris van Weel *emeritus professor of general practice*[1][2], Ryuki Kassai *professor of family medicine*[3]

[1]Department of Primary and Community Care, Radboud University Medical Center, Nijmegen, Netherlands; [2]Department of Health Services Research and Policy, Australian National University, Canberra, Australia; [3]Department of Community and Family Medicine, Fukushima Medical University, Fukushima, Japan

More than 60% of the world population live in Asia, with substantial numbers in very deprived socioeconomic conditions. The heterogeneity between the countries of the region is reflected in their health systems, which vary from well developed to virtually absent. Providing access to care, in particular for those at greatest need, is a regional priority[1] that comes on top the more general global challenge of transforming health systems to respond better to the needs of ageing populations with chronic health problems and increasing health costs.[2]

Health systems based on primary care have been shown to achieve better equity and better population health at lower costs.[3][5] Patients with chronic conditions in countries with strong primary healthcare are more likely to be in good or very good health than those in countries with less well developed primary care.[6] The same is true for frail patients with multiple chronic conditions.[7][9] This evidence has led to a global strategy to strengthen primary care,[10][11] focusing on introducing comprehensive, continuity of care in a person and population centred approach[12][13] under prevailing local conditions.[14]

Primary healthcare has to be built from the community where it has to operate, so knowledge of population needs and the existing health system is important in initiating reforms. However, most of the available experience and insight come from Europe and North America,[15][16] with data for many other many countries and regions, including South and East Asia scarce.[17] The World Organisation of Family Doctors (WONCA) therefore took the initiative to document how primary care is organised around the world and to create discussion about how the values of primary care can be adopted within the constraints of different healthcare systems.[18] This article focuses on the findings from two recent workshops at WONCA conferences in the Asia Pacific (2015)[19] and South Asia (2016)[20] regions, which critically appraised the health systems of Bangladesh, China (Shanghai region), Hong Kong, India, Japan, Nepal, Pakistan, Republic of Korea (South Korea), Singapore, Sri Lanka, and Taiwan.

Health systems in South and East Asia

The countries considered varied substantially in socioeconomic viability and in history and development of their health systems. But despite these differences, all countries were trying to strength primary healthcare. The main drivers of this policy were rising healthcare costs and the demographic changes of ageing populations with an increase of chronic health problems and multimorbidity.

In general, there is over-reliance on the hospital setting as the main provider of care and poor coordination between the hospital and community health services. This was true even in countries with developed primary care systems (Singapore, Shanghai-China, Hong Kong, and Sri Lanka). The teaching and training of health professionals—and in particular of physicians—takes place virtually exclusively in hospitals, with a strong focus on specialisation and a lack of recognition and understanding of the importance of generalist professional skills and competencies.

In most health systems the private sector, with direct out-of-pocket payment, played an important role.

Implementation of primary care policy

From the country descriptions and discussions, we determined four themes that are key to determining the outcome of primary care reforms: policy setting to plan a long term process of system change; leadership of primary healthcare professionals; finance and access; and multidisciplinary approach directed at health needs in the population.

Policy setting

Implementation of primary healthcare requires a policy to secure access to healthcare at the community level in conjunction with measures to guarantee that the policy is enacted. This means provision of community based healthcare facilities, the development of primary healthcare teams, and training professionals to deal with the prevailing health problems and

Correspondence to: C van Weel chris.vanweel@radboudumc.nl

BMJ 2017;356:j634 doi: 10.1136/bmj.j634 (Published 2017 February 27)

needs in the community and the expectations that come with them.

Singapore and Shanghai-China exemplified this in their primary health policies, which are currently working to introduce a listing of patients with community practices and a primary healthcare gatekeeping function[19] in combination with investment in community facilities, team development, and teaching and training. In other countries policy regulation is either absent, haphazard, or disconnected from strategic planning to implement these regulations in the community.

Primary care leadership

Professional leadership is required to translate policy into daily practice in the community. A critical mass of trained primary healthcare professionals is therefore essential, but achieving it is made difficult by the subordinate position of primary healthcare to hospital specialists and hospital care oriented medical schools. Furthermore, even though most countries provide training in primary care, non-specialised doctors and hospital specialists can continue to practise in the community, directly accessible by patients. This may support the reallocation of care from the hospital to the community, but primary care is more than that—it means the transformation of care focused on disease management to person or population centred care, including prevention and promotion of health.

Finance and access

In most of the countries physicians' incomes are based on items of service delivered (consultations and interventions) and often include direct out-of-pocket payment by the patient. This forms a barrier to transforming care because it stimulates disease oriented interventions and hampers access—in particular, for poor people, who often have the greatest health needs. To realise equity it is important to provide universal health coverage. However, in India and Bangladesh, particularly, there is resistance to this concept in society.

Multidisciplinary approach

A multidisciplinary approach is needed to meet the broad range of health problems (from physical to mental and social) in the community and the scope of responses that have to be provided (from support, advice, and health education to preventive, diagnostic, and therapeutic interventions). Sri Lanka, Singapore, and Shanghai-China have all established multidisciplinary teams to provide primary healthcare but other countries are relying on single handed practices, which impede a broad response to the health needs in the community, including to social determinants of health. A related barrier is the cultural-societal value placed on authority, which favours specialists over generalists.[21 22] This stands in the way of a bottom-up process.

The needs of the large numbers of poor people are especially important when considering how to strengthen primary healthcare. Connecting it to universal health coverage is therefore attractive.[1 23] The rationale is that the countries that do not have strong primary healthcare at the heart of their health systems are unable to capitalise on the equitable and cost effective care that it provides.[24]

Future development

Development of primary healthcare is on the political agenda of all countries that we examined, but they vary in their success in implementing the policy. There is therefore scope for regional collaboration and exchange of experiences. Although our

analysis is based on only 11 countries of the region, it provides good information on their policies. From this perspective we make the following recommendations for regional collaboration and action.

- Health policy should aim to move healthcare out of the hospital and into the community and to shift care from disease centred to person or population centred care. To guarantee equity, access to healthcare for all—universal health coverage[1]—and reduction of out-of-pocket payment should form an integral part of this policy.

- Provision of primary healthcare should be restricted to professionals who have been trained in specific primary care competencies and skills. This will require reform of medical schools to support primary healthcare in the medical curriculum, specialty training, and research.

- Professional primary healthcare leadership is required to push for the development of primary healthcare and guide its implementation at community level. Regional and international collaboration can support the building of leadership capacity to overcome primary care's subordinate position to hospital specialists. Models of success in other countries will show policy makers, educators, specialists, community leaders, patients, and other stakeholders the potential of primary care leadership and serve as a beacon for professionals to identify with. It is important to reflect the multidisciplinary nature of primary healthcare by including nurses, midwifes, and allied health professionals.

- Leadership capacity building should be closely linked to medical schools and the healthcare education setting to make sure that primary healthcare professionals can be trained in the community under local health (care) conditions. This is as much a challenge as an opportunity to address the urban-rural divide, so prevalent in many Asian countries, by giving rural communities currently deprived of healthcare a central position in the training of health professionals and build links to universities and medical schools. This collaboration can also support primary healthcare professionals in mastering the research skills to collect data on the population under their care to create a "community diagnosis"—an understanding of the most important health problems and (social) determinants of health that warrant priority action in that community.

- Participation of patients and communities as stakeholders at the local level is an important factor in establishing community needs, but in general there is no tradition in Asia of patient or community participation. Development of strategies to give patients and communities a voice must therefore be included at the start of the reform process.

International collaboration has an important role in health reform, through advocacy of policy development and support on the ground. Such collaboration is well developed in South East Asia with the WHO regional office having a clear strategy to pursue universal health coverage through primary healthcare[1] and the participation of more and more countries in WONCA. The platforms WHO and WONCA provide for regional collaboration can therefore help implement primary healthcare policy.

Contributors and sources: Both authors have a long experience in developing primary healthcare through international comparisons and exchanges. CvW has been president of WONCA and published widely on primary healthcare research, RK has promoted primary healthcare in Japan to direct health reforms, through the presentation of best practices from around the world. Both authors prepared the two WONCA

BMJ 2017;356:j634 doi: 10.1136/bmj.j634 (Published 2017 February 27)

ANALYSIS

Summary points

Most countries in Asia are struggling to implement primary healthcare

Primary healthcare receives low investment and education compared with hospital based specialties

Joint action between policy makers, professionals, educators, community leaders, and service users is required to draw health facilities to local communities, train professionals in the local setting, and retain them in community services

Regional and international collaboration can provide models of success and advocacy for the role and function of primary healthcare

workshops and analysed and reported their findings, that formed the basis of this article. CvW developed the outline of the paper and wrote the first draft and final version. RK commented on the outline of the paper and contributed to the first draft in developing its final form.

Competing interests: We have read and understood BMJ policy on declaration of interests and have no relevant interests to declare.

Provenance and peer review: Not commissioned; externally peer reviewed.

1   WHO South East Asia Region. Resolution on strengthening community based health care service delivery. SEA/RC68/2015. 2015.

2   World Bank. Live long and prosper: aging in East Asia and Pacific. 2016. https://openknowledge.worldbank.org/handle/10986/23133

3   Starfield B. Is primary care essential? Lancet 1994;356:1129-33. doi:10.1016/S0140-6736(94)90634-3 pmid:7934497.

4   Macinko J, Starfield B, Shi L. The contribution of primary care systems to health outcomes within Organization for Economic Cooperation and Development (OECD) countries, 1970-1998. Health Serv Res 2003;356:831-65. doi:10.1111/1475-6773.00149 pmid:12822915.

5   Starfield B, Shi L, Macinko J. Contribution of primary care to health systems and health. Milbank Q 2005;356:457-502. doi:10.1111/j.1468-0009.2005.00409.x pmid:16202000.

6   Hansen J, Groenewegen PP, Boerma WG, Kringos DS. Living in a country with a strong primary care system is beneficial to people with chronic conditions. Health Aff (Millwood) 2015;356:1531-7. doi:10.1377/hlthaff.2015.0582 pmid:26355055.

7   Turner G, Clegg A. British Geriatrics Society Age UK Royal College of General Practioners. Best practice guidelines for the management of frailty: a British Geriatrics Society, Age UK and Royal College of General Practitioners report. Age Ageing 2014;356:744-7. doi:10.1093/ageing/afu138 pmid:25336440.

8   Frank C, Wilson CR. Models of primary care for frail patients. Can Fam Physician 2015;356:601-6.pmid:26380850.

9   Eklund K, Wilhelmson K, Gustafsson H, Landahl S, Dahlin-Ivanoff S. One-year outcome of frailty indicators and activities of daily living following the randomised controlled trial: "Continuum of care for frail older people". BMC Geriatr 2013;356:76. doi:10.1186/1471-2318-13-76 pmid:23875866.

10   World Health Organization. The world health report 2008—primary health care, now more than ever. 2008. http://www.who.int/whr/2008/en/

11   World Health Assembly. 2009. Resolution 62.12 Primary health care, including health system strengthening. http://apps.who.int/gb/ebwha/pdf_files/WHA62-REC1/WHA62_REC1-en.pdf

12   Reeve J, Blakeman T, Freeman GK, et al. Generalist solutions to complex problems: generating practice-based evidence—the example of managing multi-morbidity. BMC Fam Pract 2013;356:112. doi:10.1186/1471-2296-14-112 pmid:23919296.

13   WONCA Europe. The European definition of general practice/family medicine. http://www.woncaeurope.org/sites/default/files/documents/Definition%203rd%20ed%202011%20with%20revised%20wonca%20tree.pdf

14   Kidd M, ed. The contribution of family medicine to improving health systems. A guidebook from the World Organization of Family Doctors. 2nd ed. Radcliffe Publishing, 2013.

15   J Am Board Fam Med 2012;356(suppl 1). http://www.jabfm.org/content/25/Suppl_1.toc

16   Kringos D. The strength of primary care in Europe. Thesis, University of Utrecht, 2012. http://www.nivel.nl/sites/default/files/bestanden/Proefschrift-Dionne-Kringos-The-strength-of-primary-care.pdf

17   van Weel C, Turnbull D, Whitehead E, et al. International collaboration in innovating health systems. Ann Fam Med 2015;356:86-7. doi:10.1370/afm.1751 pmid:25583898.

18   WONCA Research Working Party. Multi-national plenary panel project. http://www.globalfamilydoctor.com/groups/WorkingParties/Research/plenarypanelprojectresourcedocuments.aspx

19   van Weel C, Kassai R, Tsoi GWW, et al. Evolving health policy for primary care in the Asia Pacific region. Br J Gen Pract 2016;356:e451-3. doi:10.3399/bjgp16X685513 pmid:27231305.

20   van Weel C, Kassai R, Qidwai W, et al. Primary health care policy implementation in South Asia.BMJ Global Health 2016;356:e000057. doi:10.1136/bmjgh-2016-000057.

21   Javanparast S, Coveney J, Saikia U. Exploring health stakeholders' perceptions on moving towards comprehensive primary health care to address childhood malnutrition in Iran: a qualitative study. BMC Health Serv Res 2009;356:36. doi:10.1186/1472-6963-9-36 pmid:19236720.

22   Kassai R. Primary care and the integrated community care system in Japan: roles and future tasks [in Japanese]. Jpn J Health Economic Policy 2014;26:3-26.

23   Jha A, Godlee F, Abbasi K. Delivering on the promise of universal health coverage. BMJ 2016;356:i2216. doi:10.1136/bmj.i2216 pmid:27117561.

24   Stigler FL, Macinko J, Pettigrew LM, Kumar R, van Weel C. No universal health coverage without primary health care. Lancet 2016;356:1811. doi:10.1016/S0140-6736(16)30315-4 pmid:27203497.

Attribution

Weel C van, Kassai R. Expanding primary care in South and East Asia. *BMJ* 2017;356:j634. doi: 10.1136/bmj.j634. Reproduced with permission.

CHAPTER 16

Analysis of South–South collaboration in Africa

Maaike Flinkenflögel, Akye Essuman, Patrick Chege, Olayinka Ayankogbe and Jan De Maeseneer

Family Practice Advance Access published May 23, 2014

Family Practice, 2014, Vol. 00, No. 00, 1–10
doi:10.1093/fampra/cmu014

Family medicine training in sub-Saharan Africa: South–South cooperation in the Primafamed project as strategy for development

Maaike Flinkenflögel[a,b,]*, Akye Essuman[c,Ψ], Patrick Chege[d,Ψ], Olayinka Ayankogbe[e,Ψ] and Jan De Maeseneer[b]

[a]Department of Family and Community Medicine (FAMCO), National University of Rwanda, Butare, Rwanda, [b]Department of Family Medicine and PHC, Ghent University, Ghent, Belgium, [c]Department of Community Health, University of Ghana, Accra, Ghana, [d]Division of Family Medicine, Moi University, Eldoret, Kenya and [e]Department of Community Health and Primary Care, University of Lagos, Lagos, Nigeria.

*Correspondence to Dr Maaike Flinkenflögel, Rwinkwavu Hospital, Partners In Health, PO Box 3432, Kacyiru Sud, World Vision Street, Kigali, Rwanda; E-mail: maaike.cotc@gmail.com
[Ψ]Equal contributors.

Received August 13 2013; revised February 10 2014; Accepted March 20 2014.

Abstract

Background. Health-care systems based on primary health care (PHC) are more equitable and cost effective. Family medicine trains medical doctors in comprehensive PHC with knowledge and skills that are needed to increase quality of care. Family medicine is a relatively new specialty in sub-Saharan Africa.

Objective. To explore the extent to which the Primafamed South–South cooperative project contributed to the development of family medicine in sub-Saharan Africa.

Methods. The Primafamed (Primary Health Care and Family Medicine Education) project worked together with 10 partner universities in sub-Saharan Africa to develop family medicine training programmes over a period of 2.5 years. A SWOT (strengths, weaknesses, opportunities and threats) analysis was done and the training development from 2008 to 2010 in the different partner universities was analysed.

Results. During the 2.5 years of the Primafamed project, all partner universities made progress in the development of their family medicine training programmes. The SWOT analysis showed that at both national and international levels, the time is ripe to train medical doctors in family medicine and to integrate the specialty into health-care systems, although many barriers, including little awareness, lack of funding, low support from other specialists and reserved support from policymakers, are still present.

Conclusions. Family medicine can play an important role in health-care systems in sub-Saharan Africa; however, developing a new discipline is challenging. Advocacy, local ownership, action research and support from governments are necessary to develop family medicine and increase its impact. The Primafamed project showed that development of sustainable family medicine training programmes is a feasible but slow process. The South–South cooperation between the ten partners and the South African departments of family medicine strengthened confidence at both national and international levels.

Key words: Continuing medical education (CME), faculty development, family health, graduate medical education/fellowship training, international health.

Family Practice, 2014, Vol. 00, No. 00

Introduction

Health systems based on primary health care (PHC) distribute health care more equitably, are more cost effective and have better overall health outcomes and impact than health systems based on specialist care (1). This is the foundation of the 'Health for All' concept of Alma-Ata, adopted by the World Health Organization (WHO) in 1978 (2) and reiterated in the World Health Report 2008 (3). Worldwide, authorities have recognized that the health and well-being of a population is highly dependent on a quality PHC system that is equitable, easily accessible and affordable for all members of the community (4) and that emphasizes universal coverage (5).

The concept of the postgraduate-trained family physician qualified to deliver equitable, high-quality PHC closer to the community is now accepted in many countries around the world. However, in sub-Saharan Africa, family medicine is still a relatively new concept. In this article, we analyse the development of family medicine in Anglophone sub-Saharan Africa in the recent years based on the experiences of the Primafamed (Primary Health Care and Family Medicine Education) project (6).

Primary health care and family medicine in Africa

Lower-resource countries in sub-Saharan Africa face enormous health challenges and pervasive poverty. Despite the work of governments and nongovernmental organizations (NGOs), the majority of people still do not have easy access to affordable quality health care. The 'inverse care law' (7), noting that the fewest health-care professionals are found where they are needed the most and vice versa, is still very much applicable in most African countries. The poor are not only more prone to illnesses but are also unable to cope with diseases because health care is hard to access. With continuous population growth and a rather slow economic development, the number of people living in poverty in sub-Saharan Africa has also increased, with 20.6% living on less than US$1.25 a day in 2008 (8).

The Alma Ata Declaration was the first international statement underlining the importance of PHC. It defined PHC as part of a strategy to attain the goal of 'health for all by the year 2000' (2). It is the first level of contact of a continuing health-care process bringing health care as close as possible to where people live and work (9). PHC responds to the immense challenges that African countries are facing in their health systems by providing accessible, high-quality services that offer comprehensive and continuous care (preventive, curative, rehabilitative and palliative) at the local level, through interdisciplinary teams integrating vertical disease-oriented programmes. Family physicians together with PHC nurses (and in some countries, mid-level care workers) act as the clinical practitioners of the PHC team. In 2009, the 62nd World Health Assembly urged its member states to train and retain adequate numbers of health workers, including family physicians, and to encourage the implementation of vertical programmes in the context of integrated PHC (10).

In 1968, the University of Pretoria was the first university in South Africa to start training specialized PHC physicians, now referred to as 'African family physicians' (11). This was followed by the other seven Health Science faculties in South Africa. In 1997, these eight departments of family medicine formed a network for communication and consultation, FaMEC (Family Medicine Educational Consortium), to share and exchange expertise, form a core curriculum and standardize examinations and develop appropriate assessment systems (12). In August 2007, the South African government officially recognized family medicine as a specialty (13).

The concept of the African family physician in other Anglophone African countries is even more recent. Only in the 21st century did universities in Anglophone countries in sub-Saharan Africa start family medicine training programmes, and the recently graduated African family physicians are beginning to find their place in the health systems of their respective countries. Family medicine departments are struggling for recognition as health systems are still dominated by centralized specialist services and vertical disease-oriented approaches. Several countries, such as Namibia and Botswana, did not have medical schools until very recently (14). Furthermore, many countries, such as the Democratic Republic of Congo (DR Congo), are emerging from conflict and need to rebuild both state and infrastructure. At the WONCA (World Organisation of Family Doctors) Africa Conference in 2009, the Statement of Consensus on Family Medicine in Africa was agreed upon. This consensus statement defined the contribution of family medicine to equity, quality and PHC within an African context, as well as the role and training requirements of the African family physician (15). Due to the low number of trained doctors per capita and the high burden of disease, African family physicians work in their specific context, mainly in district hospitals with outreach to health centres, in PHC teams that address the problems of the community in a comprehensive, holistic and patient-centred way whereby specific skills like surgery and district management often are essential due to the lack of other specialists. The consensus illustrates the ownership of the development of family medicine by African universities, one of the key points from the Paris Declaration (2005) and the Accra Agenda for Action (2008) (16).

Objectives

The aim of this article is to explore the extent to which the Primafamed South–South cooperative project contributed to the development of family medicine in sub-Saharan Africa. The specific objectives are the following:

1. The implementation of the Primafamed project;
2. The outcomes of the Primafamed project;
3. The development of family medicine training in sub-Saharan Africa from the viewpoint of the Primafamed partners.

Methods

A process analysis of the Primafamed project between 2008 and 2011 is presented to discuss the implementation of the programme and the development of the network of 10 universities and associated partners in Anglophone sub-Saharan Africa. The outcomes and conclusions of the project after 2.5 years are described. Finally, a SWOT analysis is detailed to explore the positive and negative dynamics that partners faced during the project.

The Primafamed Edulink project

In 2007, a call for proposals under the name Edulink was launched by the Secretariat of the African, Caribbean and Pacific (ACP) Group of States (17). Together with 10 universities in eight countries in sub-Saharan Africa (Sudan, Ghana, Nigeria, DR Congo, Rwanda, Uganda, Kenya and Tanzania), Figure 1, the Department of Family Medicine and PHC at Ghent University in Belgium developed the Primafamed project proposal with a focus on developing family medicine training in sub-Saharan Africa. The objectives of the project are described in Box 1. The aim of the Primafamed project was to establish an institutional network between new and established departments of family medicine in universities in sub-Saharan Africa, within a framework of South–South cooperation (18). The WHO World Health Report 2006, 'Working together for

health', emphasized the need for PHC training in the local community in order to deal with the brain drain from ACP states (19). Training medical doctors in the field of family medicine, thus providing PHC at the district level, responds to this call.

The Primafamed partners

The partnering universities in the Primafamed project were University of Goma (DR Congo), Moi University (Kenya), National University of Rwanda, Aga Khan University (Tanzania), University of Lagos (Nigeria), Makerere University (Uganda), Mbarara University (Uganda), Ahfad University for Women (Sudan), Gezira University (Sudan) and University of Ghana. The South–South network connecting these 10 universities worked together with the eight departments of family medicine in South Africa and accordingly formed a forum to share knowledge, experiences and resources.

Outcomes of the Primafamed project

Each of the 10 partner universities hired a local coordinator to oversee the implementation of the project, coordinate the activities and actively communicate with all partners. Partners worked independently, integrating the Primafamed objectives and the output for the project into the already existing structures and work plan at their universities. Because African family physicians work mainly in district hospitals with outreach to the health centres, this is where the bulk of family medicine training takes place. The Primafamed project consequently stimulated all partners to develop training complexes (mainly district hospitals, several of which are located in rural areas) for family medicine residents and to support the supply

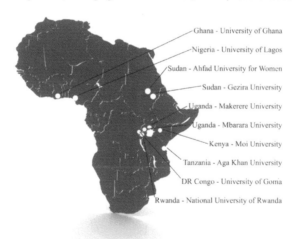

Ghana - University of Ghana

Nigeria - University of Lagos

Sudan - Ahfad University for Women

Sudan - Gezira University

Uganda - Makerere University

Uganda - Mbarara University

Kenya - Moi University

Tanzania - Aga Khan University

DR Congo - University of Goma

Rwanda - National University of Rwanda

Figure 1. The Primafamed partners. Adapted from Shutterstock.

Box 1. Objectives of the Primafamed project

The objectives of the Primafamed project were formulated as follows:

1. To contribute to the health of communities through accessible, responsive and quality health systems in sub-Saharan countries by educating and training family physicians who provide interdisciplinary PHC services, oriented towards the needs of individuals, their families and the communities in which they live.
2. To plan, develop and strengthen academic departments or units of family medicine that offer family medicine training at the undergraduate and postgraduate levels.

The specific objectives were as follows:

1. To develop a comprehensive vision and strategy, within the specific context of sub-Saharan countries, that delineates the integral contribution of family medicine and the PHC team to an equitable and quality PHC system;
2. To establish a specific institutional network between departments and units of family medicine.

The expected results of the Primafamed project were the following:

1. An improved institutional and administrative functioning in terms of policy, management, planning and administrative capacity building of the participating departments and units of family medicine.
2. Improved relevance of family medicine in undergraduate and postgraduate training in the regional context.
3. Research output with respect to curriculum development in family medicine.

Box 2. Progress scale for development of the Primafamed partners

Level 1:
  – Structural implementation of the training programme and the department is in preparation

Level 2:
  – Department/unit of family medicine exists or is part of other departments (community medicine)
  – Training complexes are under development
  – Family medicine is part of undergraduate training

Level 3:
  – Department/unit of family medicine exists
  – Training complexes are in place
  – Curriculum is written
  – Postgraduate training has started

Level 4:
  – Department/unit of family medicine exists
  – Training complexes are in place
  – Curriculum is written
  – Postgraduate training has started
  – The Ministry of Health has accepted family medicine as a specialization and graduated family physicians are part of the health-care systemAdopted from the Primafamed Edulink ACP EU project.

---

of these training complexes with the needed equipment. To further strengthen family medicine residents' education, training sessions by professors from South African universities and other associated Primafamed partners were held. A yearly conference for partners, associates and stakeholders was organized with the goal of offering trainings, sharing ideas and experiences, and strengthening the network. At the 2008 conference in Kampala, the *African Journal of Primary Health Care and Family Medicine* (20) was launched. This new open-access online journal has since published various articles related to the development of family medicine on the African continent, and researchers in the field of PHC have written numerous articles on operational research and community-oriented primary care (COPC) projects (21).

To monitor and evaluate our project, a progress scale was developed (Box 2). This four-level scale shows the progress that took place during the 2.5-year period in which Primafamed supported the partners. The first level corresponds to the institution being at a preparatory stage in the development of a postgraduate family medicine training programme. The fourth level reflects that the institution has started a postgraduate family medicine training programme with an existing curriculum by an organized department at well-organized training complexes and, most importantly, that family medicine has been accepted by the Ministry of Health as a specialization and that graduated family physicians are integrated into the existing health system. Undeniably, the fourth level is not the end stage because, in our opinion, the ultimate objective would be to have an equitable and high-quality PHC system with a central role for family physicians.

All 10 Primafamed partners made progress during the 2.5 years that the project provided funding and support (Table 1). At the start of the project, all of them had a unit or department of family medicine under development or in place, yet only three had officially started postgraduate family medicine training. At the end of the project, eight had started postgraduate training, with family medicine residents located in properly equipped training hospitals.

Table 1. Progress scale for development of the Primafamed partners

	January 2008, start of the Primafamed project	July 2010, end of the Primafamed project
University of Goma, DRC	Level 2	Level 4
Moi University, Kenya	Level 3	Level 4
National University of Rwanda	Level 2	Level 4
Aga Khan University, Tanzania	Level 2	Level 3
University of Lagos, Nigeria	Level 1	Level 2
Makerere University, Uganda	Level 3	Level 3
Mbarara University, Uganda	Level 2	Level 3
Ahfad University for Women, Sudan	Level 1	Level 2
Gezira University, Sudan	Level 1	Level 4
University of Ghana	Level 3	Level 4

Adopted from the Primafamed Edulink ACP-EU project.

The integration of family medicine into the local health systems has been a slower process. In many countries, policymakers have adopted a somewhat conservative attitude, with health systems mainly based on hospital/specialist care and on vertical programmes, which are often stimulated by donor programmes. A critical mass of well-trained family physicians is needed to demonstrate the effectiveness of family medicine training programmes. Because all but one partner universities train only a limited number of family medicine residents simultaneously due to limited capacity, reaching that critical mass takes time. However, as the example of Gezira University (Sudan) has shown, it is possible to create a large pool of well-trained family physicians who can make a difference, in a short time. In this particular situation, because there was a vital need, policymakers and local authorities worked closely together with Gezira University in development of the training (Example 1).

In 2012, African family physicians came together at the WONCA Africa Conference and the Primafamed Network Workshop in Victoria Falls, Zimbabwe, and reaffirmed the importance of reaching that critical mass and therefore scaling up of family medicine, particularly in the African context, in which poverty is very prevalent, where rural–urban gaps remain, and where many of the Millennium Development Goals (MDGs) will not be reached, including those related to child survival, maternal death and accessibility to antiretroviral drugs (22).

SWOT analysis

In 2010, all Primafamed local coordinators contributed to a SWOT (strengths, weaknesses, opportunities and threats) analysis on the development of family medicine training programmes and of family medicine as a new discipline within the health systems of their countries (Box 3). The main findings are presented

Box 3. SWOT analysis of family medicine training in the Primafamed partnering countries

Strengths
- Strong partnerships and collaboration with universities and professional bodies abroad is present
- The South African departments of family medicine have substantial experience in the family medicine training programmes: they can assist in training *via* South–South cooperation and these cooperative steps can be seen as exemplary models and 'good practices'
- The Primafamed project and Edulink ACP-EU funding strengthens the development of family medicine training and is seen as the motor for the family medicine training development
- Individuals working in the family medicine departments are very motivated, proactive and willing to advocate for the cause
- Family physicians working as faculty are highly experienced and well qualified
- The chosen district hospitals and health centres are ready for the training programmes
- In several of the countries (Sudan, Kenya and Ghana), a high commitment from the Ministry of Health, the National Council and leaders is existing
- Family medicine is responsive to the needs of the communities, especially in the rural areas where the majority of Africans live

Weaknesses
- Family medicine is not yet part of undergraduate medical training, therefore medical students are not exposed to the concept of family medicine and its principles
- Poor quality of intake and recruitment of family medicine residents for the family medicine training
- The lack of family physicians and local teachers. Many of the departments of family medicine depend on family physicians coming from non-African countries (mainly, Western Europe and United States)
- Due to work overload, family medicine residents are continuously working in the hospital setting and have insufficient time to focus on the training in other aspects of family medicine, such as disease prevention and health promotion, community medicine, outpatient/continuity of care and research
- The existing health systems are still weak in several countries; plagued by poor support, weak referral systems, poor communication, poor funding and poor coordination between health centres, district hospitals and referral hospitals

Family Practice, 2014, Vol. 00, No. 00

- Dropping out of family medicine residents during the training sometimes happens in countries like DR Congo because family medicine residents lose faith in their career opportunities
- There is a lack of didactic materials
- Capacity is still too limited
- There is poor guidance for the present faculty
- There is a lack of awareness and knowledge of family medicine by medical graduates, specialists and the community
- There is lack of adequate infrastructure in some countries, such as DR Congo and Ghana
- There is poor communication with policymakers and little support from the government in countries like Tanzania and Rwanda[i]
- Standardization of training and examinations between faculties and countries is presently not existing, although there is a strong need for accreditation and quality assurance
- There is insufficient financial support for the family medicine residents in postgraduate training
- The position of family physicians in the different health systems is unclear (What is the career perspective of graduated family physicians?)

Opportunities
- There is international support for the concept of family medicine: In the World Health Report 2008 'Primary Health Care: Now more than ever', the WHO advocated for the importance of moving health care out of tertiary hospitals into the community and from vertical to horizontal care, in order to respond to the needs of the community
- Family medicine training is growing in the whole African continent, and there is support in the surrounding countries. The Primafamed project has been linking these different countries, in order to fight for the cause together
- Existing health systems in several countries are weak (poor coordination, poor referral systems, poor communication and little funding). Family medicine can be used as a technique to strengthen these health systems
- Internet connection is present in several of the training centres (and this is rapidly expanding); e-learning is a very useful didactic tool for the family medicine residents
- A yearly conference is organized by the Primafamed network to strengthen the network and to share ideas and exchange experiences
- Wonca[ii] Africa is organizing three yearly conferences and has been expanding in terms of number of members in the recent years

- There are many existing links with organizations and universities in the North for financial and didactic support
- IUCEA[iii] and WACP[iv] can assist in accreditation and quality assurance
- Several very useful books on African family medicine have been published recently and can be used as training material
- The new *African Journal of Primary Health Care and Family Medicine* gives more opportunities for registrars to publish research
- Health-care workers and policymakers are becoming increasingly aware of the importance of the basic principles of PHC and family medicine such as patient-centred care, non-communicable diseases (NCDs), interdisciplinary care, and continuity of care
- Many African ministries of health are working on health-system reforms
- Research in the field of family medicine is done by the registrars during the training
- The Primafamed network has been looking into expanding to Francophone Africa: Mali and Benin will participate in a VLIR UOS–funded project starting 2012, and the *African Journal of Primary Health Care and Family Medicine* will be published in English and French from 2012 onwards

Threats
- Other specialities see family medicine as a threat
- Family medicine is a new concept and not yet part of the health system in most of the partnering countries
- Overload of work for doctors leads to little time for training
- Lack of career opportunities for family medicine physicians in countries where family medicine is not supported by the government
- There is little or no funding for family medicine within the existing systems
- Substantial decrease in funding for further development of the family medicine training after ending of the Primafamed project funding from Edulink ACP-EU
- Migration of graduates to private practice, NGOs, management positions or public health (internal brain drain) or migration of graduates to other countries (external brain drain)[v]
- War and political instability (e.g. DR Congo, Sudan and Nigeria); in some countries, there is a high turnover of government and with this, there often is a change of policies
- Increasing commercialization and privatization of health-care provision

- – Worldwide economic crisis, which is decreasing the funding for health care and is putting health systems under pressure
- – Fragmentation of care through vertical disease-oriented programmes, not only for infectious diseases, but increasingly for NCDs (23).

i. When the SWOT analysis was done in 2010, the Rwandan Ministry of Health was supportive of the new discipline and family medicine was accepted by the government as one of the specialist MMed trainings from the National University of Rwanda. However, at the time of writing this article, the Ministry of Health in Rwanda has changed its vision and family medicine is not seen as a priority. Recently, financial support for the training was reduced.

ii. World Organisation of Family Physicians

iii. Inter-University Council of East Africa

iv. West African College of Physicians

v. Especially in Sudan, this is a problem as a large percentage of medical graduates move to Saudi Arabia for more job opportunities, better salaries or family reasons

Adopted from the Primafamed Edulink ACP EU project

and categorized into the following levels: local/university level, national level, regional/African level and international level.

At the local/university level, the availability of resources plays an important role. From a human resources perspective, family physicians (in most cases from abroad) are needed to form the faculty, train family medicine residents and develop teaching materials. Other local professors and specialists willing to train family medicine residents in the different disciplines are important to the strengthening of both the training and the interdisciplinary network; however, several partners noted a low level of support from other specialists because family medicine is often not well understood and is often seen as a threat. Adequate motivation of faculty and family medicine residents is important and is influenced by many other factors such as financial backing, career opportunities and support at the local, national and international levels. The availability of training sites, especially at district hospitals and health centres, is crucial, including having access to physicians to train and mentor the family medicine residents and stimulating teamwork with other health-care workers such as the local nurses. Well-written curricula (often developed based on sample curricula from family medicine training programmes in other African universities) and training materials are essential to create a high-quality training atmosphere. Access to the Internet and to didactic materials and equipment (such an ultrasound machines or health education materials) are important to strengthen the actual training. Lack of diagnostic or therapeutic equipments or insufficient availability of essential drugs in the training hospitals influences the way the doctors learn and hinders implementation of evidence-based medicine. Ensuring that there is a place for family medicine training in undergraduate curricula plays a crucial role in raising awareness and recruiting newly trained medical doctors.

At the national level, policymakers play a pivotal role. In several countries, decision-makers accept family medicine as an official specialization that is starting to take its place in the health-care system, with Kenya, Sudan and Ghana as examples (see Examples 1, 2 and 3). Several other countries have had more difficulties with the Ministry of Health accepting family medicine, including Tanzania and Rwanda. This influences career safety prospects for family physicians and therefore renders recruitment more difficult. Continuous communication and advocacy to create awareness and understanding are important. Research on the positive outcomes of family medicine on health-care provision plays a significant role in advocating and strengthening awareness. A negative factor at the national level is political instability and war, as seen in Eastern Congo.

At the regional/African level, the importance of strong partnerships and collaboration with universities and professional bodies abroad is noted. South African universities have excellent curricula and knowledgeable professors with extensive experience that can be leveraged *via* South–South cooperation. Moreover, conferences organized by Primafamed and WONCA Africa support the development of African family medicine. Networks are created to support each other and to start joint research. The establishment of the *African Journal of Primary Health Care and Family Medicine* is a great opportunity for young researchers to learn from others' work and to publish their own articles.

At the international level, a key point is the funding and support from institutes in the North. Secondly, global recognition of the importance of training health-care workers in PHC (World Health Report 2006 and 2008) is vital to the development of African family medicine. However, fragmentation of care undermines the importance of comprehensive PHC (23).

Conclusions

The ultimate goal of health care is to reverse the 'inverse care law' through achieving universal coverage and by providing equitable and high-quality health care through well-trained health-care workers to every individual. This is what health systems based on PHC can provide. Training doctors who work closer to communities, where they are most needed, is an important step towards improving the health outcomes of the African population. However, developing a new discipline that has not yet been defined in the national health systems is a challenging task.

The Primafamed project showed that developing sustainable family medicine training programmes is a feasible but slow

Family Practice, 2014, Vol. 00, No. 00

process with many obstacles. The South–South cooperation between the Primafamed partners and the South African family medicine departments strengthened confidence in the project and reinforced the principal need for well-trained African family physicians. Local ownership is of utmost importance, although, with no local family physicians as role models, this can be a difficult task. Support from key figures at the level of policymakers and academicians is necessary to create this new discipline and give it a place in health systems. Without the integration of family medicine into national health policy, it is very difficult to recruit new doctors for the training programmes because the uncertainty in career prospects negatively influences a potential candidate's decision to join these programmes. Continuous advocacy for the discipline and for strengthening the role of the African family physician are crucial. Exposure to family medicine and community health in the undergraduate medical curriculum is required to create awareness among new medical doctors. Action research, such as COPC (24), in the African setting is needed to demonstrate significant outcomes and the positive influence of the discipline at the individual, community and national levels. Recruitment, training and retention of doctors in family medicine need to be adopted in the health system of each of the African countries. This requires increased investment of resources in PHC, both from governments and from donor organizations.

The Primafamed Network that was created during the 2008–10 project continues to endeavour to make these action points a reality. In November 2012, during the WONCA Africa Conference, representatives from many African family medicine departments came together and discussed steps forward in creating a strong family medicine and PHC-oriented health-care system in various African countries. This led to the 'Statement of the Primafamed Network: Scaling up family medicine and primary health care in Africa'. Concrete action for scaling up is needed, including convincing ministries and leadership of medical schools to integrate family medicine and PHC into the undergraduate curriculum and to train a significant proportion of medical school graduates (between 40% and 60%) in family medicine and PHC. Essential conditions include having accredited under- and postgraduate curricula; well-equipped training centres for transformative learning with well-trained trainers; national and international support networks; a sufficient number of funded posts for family medicine residents/registrars with appropriate remuneration; and continuous advocacy at the population and government levels (25).

Continuous interaction with key players at the policymaking level and support from the government are necessary to scale up family medicine and to develop it into an essential part of the health-care systems, in order to provide equitable, high-quality

health care for communities and, ultimately, to improve overall health in sub-Saharan Africa.

Example 1. Sudanese family physicians

Gezira University is a public university based in central Sudan, in the city of Wad Madani. When the Primafamed project started, family medicine did not yet exist in Sudan. In many health centres, community physicians and medical officers were in charge of patient care. Together with policymakers, district health officers and representatives from the Ministry of Health identified the need for further training for medical doctors in Primary Health Care. Gezira University decided to develop a 1-year diploma and a 2-year in-service Master of Science (MSc) in family medicine. Both are accepted by the Sudan National Medical Specialisation Board. With the help of the Primafamed project, a coordinator for this development was financed, a curriculum was developed and training sites were identified and equipped with the needed material. In 2009–10, the first 10 medical doctors were trained in the 1-year course. In 2010, 120 candidates were selected for the 2-year in-service MSc in family medicine. In the fall of 2012, these 120 Sudanese family physicians graduated with comprehensive knowledge in district primary health care. In 2013, 200 new candidates were selected. The University of Gezira can be seen as a perfect example of how working together with policymakers is essential for the development of family medicine. Adopted from the Primafamed Edulink ACP EU final report.

Example 2. Family medicine training at Moi University, Eldoret, Kenya

In 2005, Moi University started the first family medicine training programme in Anglophone Eastern Africa, outside South Africa, Nigeria and Ghana, leading to the degree of Master of Medicine in Family Health. The development of this residency programme was a triangular effort from Moi University, Infa-Med (Institute of Family Medicine, a faith-based NGO, aiming to introduce family medicine in Kenya) and the Kenyan Ministry of Health (MoH). Moi University provided central facilities, academic leadership and long-term vision. Infa-Med contributed financial support, expatriate family medicine faculty and well-established training hospitals; and the MoH provided political support to the new specialty as well as scholarships to medical doctors entering the residency programme (26). A national policy (the Kenyan Family Medicine Policy) was developed (27) and in August 2009, this was adopted by the Kenyan government. In 2008, the first registrars finalized the family medicine programme at Moi University. Most of these registrars are now working in connection with the department to further develop the curriculum and the training sites.

A study in 2011 on the challenges of family physicians after placement showed that the ministry's posting policy needs to be improved to ensure that family physicians have a chance to perform their intended roles (28). In 2011, one of the first-graduated Kenyan family physicians, Dr Patrick Chege, became the Head of Department. The department of family medicine has strongly been focussing on the development of research. In 2009, a review of the present family medicine curriculum was started to improve the curriculum with a focus on the needs of the hospitals where the family physicians will be based. Many external experts from Primafamed partners and associates were consulted in this process. In January 2012, the revised curriculum was approved by the Moi University Senate.

Example 3. Family medicine in Ghana

The West African College of Physicians (WACP) accepted family medicine in 1985 (29) and it extended to the subregion outside Nigeria in 1991 (29). In Ghana, postgraduate training began in March 1999 with three family medicine residents under the auspices of the Faculty of Family Medicine (then General Medical Practice) of the WACP. This was a hospital-based training programme with the initial group of trainers being private general practitioners who were elected into fellowship by the College in the early 1990s. It started as a 4-year programme leading to Membership after the initial 2 years and Fellowship after a further training for 2 years. Currently, one trains for 3 years for Membership. The first graduate fellow completed training in April 2005. That same year, the Ghana College of Physicians and Surgeons also started another programme in family medicine to run alongside the one conducted by WACP. The Ministry of Health provides sponsorship for the programmes and accords graduates of family medicine equal status and remuneration as graduates from other specialties. In January 2008, the undergraduate programme began in the University of Ghana Medical School with the first two fellowship graduates appointed as lecturers. The undergraduate unit is currently part of the Department of Community Health. These local efforts at promoting the specialty in Ghana received a major boost with two significant collaborations: first with the Primafamed Edulink ACP-EU project in 2007, a North–South–South cooperation, and second, with the Department of Family Medicine, University of Michigan Health Systems in 2008, a North–South cooperation. These collaborations focussed on curriculum development, faculty development, teaching of students and family medicine residents, development of training complexes and research. Currently, there are two well-established postgraduate training complexes in Accra (Korle-Bu Teaching Hospital) and Kumasi (Komfo-Anokye Teaching Hospital) with 35 family medicine residents at various levels of membership and fellowship training (30).

Acknowledgements

MF was responsible for the conception of the research and the general outline of the article, AE, PC and OA contributed through the documentation of different parts of the article. JDM is the promoter of the Primafamed project. The manuscript was reviewed by all authors.

Declaration

Funding: The Primafamed project was funded by the Edulink ACP EU (European Commission funded programmes in the Africa, Caribbean and Pacific Group of States). The VLIR UOS (Flemish Interuniversity Council) supported the funding for the yearly Primafamed conferences—2008 in Kampala, Uganda; 2009 in Rustenburg, South Africa; 2010 in Swaziland and 2011 in Cape Town, South Africa. The authors did not receive any extra funding to write this article.
Ethical approval: No ethical approval was sought.
Conflict of interest: None of the authors reports a conflict of interest.

References

1. Starfield B, Shi L, Macinko J. Contribution of primary care to health systems and health. *Milbank Q* 2005; 83: 457–502.
2. Mahler H. The Meaning of "health for All by the Year 2000". World Health Organization; 1981 [cited 7 January 2014]. http://whqlibdoc.who.int/temp/Mahler_1981_WorldHealthForum.pdf.
3. World Health Organization, Lerberghe W van. *Primary Health Care: Now More Than Ever*. Geneva, Switzerland: World Health Organization, 2008.
4. Borisch B. Global health equity: opportunities and threats. *J Public Health Policy* 2012; 33: 488–91.
5. Discussion Paper, International Conference on Primary Health Care and Health Systems in Africa. World Health Organisation; April 2008 [cited 21 April 2014]. http://www.afro.who.int/index.php?option=com_content&view=article&id=2034&Itemid=830.
6. www.primafamed.ugent.be.
7. Tudor HJ. The inverse care law. *The Lancet* 1971; 297: 405–12.
8. World Databank. World Development Indicators & Global Development Finance [cited 22 May 2012]. www.worldbank.org/en/topic/poverty/overview.
9. Rawaf S, De Maeseneer J, Starfield B. From Alma-Ata to Almaty: a new start for primary health care. *Lancet* 2008; 372: 1365–7.
10. World Health Assembly 62.12. Geneva, Switzerland: World Health Organization; May 2009 [cited 7 January 2014]. http://www.who.int/hrh/resources/A62_12_EN.pdf.
11. Hugo J, Allen L. *Doctors for Tomorrow*. 1st edn. South Africa: NISC, 2007.
12. Training in Family Medicine and Primary Health Care in South-Africa and Flanders: report of a study visit. Belgium; September 1997. Report No.: Projectnr. ZA.96.11.
13. Hellenberg D, Gibbs T. Developing family medicine in South africa: a new and important step for medical education. *Med Teach* 2007; 29: 897–900.
14. Mash B, Downing R, Moosa S, De Maeseneer J. Exploring the key principles of Family Medicine in sub-Saharan Africa: international Delphi consensus process. *South Afr Fam Pract* 2008; 50: 60–5.
15. Mash B, Reid S. Statement of consensus on family medicine in Africa. *Afr J Prim Health Care Fam Med* 2010; 2: 4.

Family Practice, 2014, Vol. 00, No. 00

16. Paris declaration on aid effectiveness and the Accra agenda for action. Organisation for Economic Co-operation and Development. 2005/2008. [cited 7 January 2014]. www.oecd.org/development/effectiveness/34428351.pdf.

17. ACP-EU Cooperation Programme in Higher Education (EDULINK). Guidelines for grant applicants responding to the call for proposals for 2007. Edulink ACP-EU; 2007 [cited 7 January 2014]. http://programasue.info/documentos/2007-EuropeAid-125565.pdf.

18. Du Toit L. *South-South Cooperation in Health Science Education: A Literature Review.* Johannesburg: Wits Centre for Rural Health, July 2011.

19. Chen LC, World Health Organization. The world health report 2006 working together for health. Geneva: World Health Organization, 2006 [cited 7 January 2014]. www.who.int/whr/2006/whr06%5Fen.pdf.

20. African Journal of Primary Health Care and Family Medicine. *OASIS Open Journals*, 2014 [cited 21 April 2014]. www.phcfm.org.

21. African Journal of Primary Health Care and Family Medicine. Readership statistics 2009–2010. *Aosis Open Journals* 2012.

22. The Millennium Development Goals Report 2013. United Nations, 2013 [cited 14 January 2014]. www.un.org/millenniumgoals/pdf/report-2013/mdg-report-2013-english.pdf.

23. De Maeseneer J, Roberts R, Demarzo M *et al.* Tackling NCD's: a different approach is needed. *The Lancet* 2011; 6736: 61135–5.

24. Rhyne R, Bogue RJ, Kukulka G, Fulmer H. *Community Oriented Primary Care: Health Care for the 21st Century.* American Public Health Association, 1998.

25. De Maeseneer J. Scaling up Family Medicine (FM) and Primary Health Care (PHC) in Africa: statement of the Primafamed network. Victoria Falls, Zimbabwe: Primafamed Network, November 2012.

26. Pust R, Dahlman B, Khwa-Otsyula B, Armstrong J, Downing R. Partnerships creating postgraduate family medicine in Kenya. *Fam Med* 2006; 38: 661–6.

27. Kenyan Family Medicine Strategy.

28. Voort van der T, Kasteren G, Chege P, Dinant G. What challenges hamper Kenyan family physicians in pursuing their family medicine mandate? A qualitative study among family physicians and their colleagues. *BMC Fam Pract* 2012; 13: 32.

29. Binitie A, Acquaye J. *History of the West African College of Physicians 1972–2000.* WACP, 2010.

30. Annual faculty report 2011. Faculty of Family Medicine, Ghana College of Physicians and Surgeons, 2011.

Attribution

Flinkenflögel M, Essuman A, Chege P, Ayankogbe O, De Maeseneer J. Family medicine training in sub-Saharan Africa: South–South cooperation in the Primafamed project as strategy for development. *Family Practice* 2014;31:427–436. doi: 10.1093/fampra/cmu014. Reproduced with permission.

CHAPTER 17

Coping with political scepticism

Chris van Weel, Deborah Turnbull, Andrew Bazemore, Carmen Garcia-Penã, Martin Roland, Richard H. Glazier, Robert L. Phillips and Felicity Goodyear-Smith

FAMILY MEDICINE UPDATES

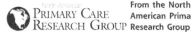

From the North American Primary Care Research Group

Ann Fam Med 2018;16:179-180. https://doi.org/10.1370/afm.2214.

IMPLEMENTING PRIMARY HEALTH CARE POLICY UNDER CHANGING GLOBAL POLITICAL CONDITIONS: LESSONS LEARNED FROM 4 NATIONAL SETTINGS

Based on the International Workshop at the NAP-CRG Conference in Colorado Springs, November 13, 2016, a full report is published at http://bit.do/NAPCRGFullPaperImplementingPrimaryHealthcare.

Health systems struggle with equitable and affordable health spending. Over-medication, low-value care, poor access and social determinants of health amplify inequity. At the same time, primary health care (PHC) improves efficiency, equity, effectiveness, and population health. Community-based–person- and population-centered care reduces health inequalities. This requires ongoing policy. This paper explores how to secure long-term PHC policies, from policy makers obsessed with "quick wins."

Appealing to Policy Makers

Investment in PHC reduces inefficiency and/or overall costs. Studies reported a 43% increase in PHC spending resulted in a 14% reduction in total health spending; yielded a 13-fold return on this investment; and improved the effectiveness and efficiency of the health system. Yet, this does not guarantee policy makers' commitment. Too often, experiments are prematurely abandoned: for example in Brazil, where PHC was associated with reduced hospitalization; or in the United States, where PHC reduced costs and hospitalizations but rapid consolidation of PHC policy restricted comprehensiveness.

Social inequities affect a range of outcomes from life expectancy, crime, education, and mental health. Greater equality has the strongest impact for the poorest, but also benefits those socioeconomically well-off. This should encourage policy makers to address social determinants of health through PHC as an affordable, politically attractive solution. In this context, experiences from the United Kingdom, Canada, Mexico, and the United States are presented.

Experiences

England

A crisis in general practice, caused by an increased workload, poor recruitment, and mounting early retirement, was the "tipping point" for major policy changes. A report was commissioned that contained 38 mainly uncontentious, earlier argued-for recommendations. This resulted in the adoption of major increases in funding and staffing (http://bit.do/NAPCRGFullPaperImplementingPrimaryHealthcare). It took a developing crisis and professional consensus to produce action by government.

Canada

Canada's primary care physician shortage and poor rankings on international comparisons persuaded policy makers to invest in PHC. Transformation of the health system was done with emphasis on PHC payment reforms, inter-professional teams, after-hours access, electronic health record systems, regionalization, and development of clinical networks. This increased the PHC workforce, including many non-physicians. Pilot projects and local initiatives improved outcomes, but had limited scale and impact. This restricted PHC's contribution to population health, patient experience and costs—due to continued fee-for-service payments, and poor integration with social and community sectors and hospital care.

Mexico

The Mexican health system remains fragmented and universal coverage for PHC is not (yet) achieved. Although it is argued that PHC is at the center of the system, and family medicine specialization was introduced in 1971, pervasive inequalities persist. Main advances have been seen in reduced infant mortality and increased health promotion. In 2004 further PHC innovations were installed, but they lacked continuity of policy support for success. Population demographics (46% are aged under 25 years) remains a challenge. With uncertain commitment of politicians, insurers, and educators, advocacy of the role of PHC and patients' experiences is a priority.

United States

International comparisons of countries and health systems were important to support US policy makers in health reforms. Following this, experts from Australia, Denmark, the Netherlands, and New Zealand addressed key US policy makers about innovations in their countries: the *Embassy Conversation Series*. US responders translated this evidence from other countries into implications for the United States. After summary presentations in the US Congress, $1 billion support for research and demonstration projects was provided under the Affordable Care Act. A US-Canada *Cross-National Implementation Science Symposium* canvassed best practices in addressing multimorbidity, alternative payment models, and health equity.

The lessons that could be learned were "translated" to the US context.

International Comparisons

Findings from other developed and mainly developing countries were placed against these experiences. In general, PHC was associated with improved efficiency, access, and equity. Lessons learned were the need for consistent PHC policy over time that includes regulations on professional training, and on access to practice, while pursuit of universal health coverage creates opportunities for PHC.

Conclusions

From this, it is recommended to:

- Make sure that policy makers understand the benefits of PHC, and *how* it improves individuals' and populations' health
- Seize moments of crises in health systems to promote PHC
- Connect PHC implementation with the World Health Organization (WHO)'s universal health coverage agenda
- Engage with community leaders, policy makers, and other stakeholders in driving reforms and innovations
- Emphasize that the whole of society benefits from PHC, not only the marginalized or wealthy
- Stress that PHC development is a continuous and not a one-off process of meeting evolving needs of populations

*Chris van Weel, Radboud University Nijmegen,
The Netherlands, Australian National University, Canberra,
Australia; Deborah Turnbull, University of Adelaide,
Australia; Andrew Bazemore, Robert Graham Center Policy
Studies in Family Medicine & Primary Care,
Washington DC, USA; Carmen Garcia-Penã, National
Institute of Geriatrics, Mexico City, Mexico; Martin Roland,
Department of Public Health and Primary Care, University
of Cambridge, UK; Richard H. Glazier, Institute for
Clinical Evaluative Sciences and St. Michaels Hospital
and University of Toronto, Toronto, Canada; Robert L.
Phillips, American Board of Family Medicine,
Lexington, KY, USA; Felicity Goodyear-Smith, Department
of General Practice and Primary Health Care, University of
Auckland, Auckland, New Zealand.
(Full list at: http://bit.do/NAPCRGFull
PaperImplementingPrimaryHealthcare)*

Attribution

Weel C van, Turnbull D, Bazemore A, Garcia-Penã C, Roland M, Glazier RH, Phillips RL, Goodyear-Smith F. Implementing primary health care policy under changing global political conditions: Lessons learned from 4 national settings. *Annals of Family Medicine* 2018;16:179–180. https://doi.org/10.1370/afm.2214. Reproduced with permission.

CHAPTER 18

Primary health care to contribute to universal health coverage

Chris van Weel and Michael R. Kidd

ANALYSIS ▌▌ HEALTH SERVICES

Why strengthening primary health care is essential to achieving universal health coverage

Chris van Weel MD PhD, Michael R. Kidd AM

▪ Cite as: *CMAJ* 2018 April 16;190:E463-6. doi: 10.1503/cmaj.170784

See related article at www.cmaj.ca/lookup/doi/10.1503/cmaj.180186

S trengthening primary health care[1] and the attainment of universal health coverage[2,3] are both important current global health policy initiatives. Primary health care is essential and affordable care that is accessible to everyone in the community, and includes health promotion, disease prevention, health maintenance, education and rehabilitation.[4] The concept of universal health coverage, as noted in the United Nations' 2015 Sustainable Development Goals, is an aspiration to provide all people with access to essential high-quality health services and to safe, effective and affordable medicines and vaccines, while ensuring financial risk protection by providing care regardless of a person's ability to pay for it.[2,5] It is clear from these two definitions that there is overlap between the aims of primary health care and universal health coverage; indeed, many have noted that primary health care is essential to achieving universal coverage.[6,7]

The two agendas have developed largely independently of each other, and yet the goal of both is to see healthier people living in healthier communities. There seems to be a natural synergy between the two. Yet the World Bank, the Bill and Melinda Gates Foundation and the World Health Organization (WHO) have referred to primary health care as a "black box" for policy-makers[8] — complex, mysterious and difficult to understand. Many health care policy-makers and funders have a poor understanding of primary health care, finding it difficult to quantify and assess its contributions to health systems. Here, we shine a light into the "black box." We emphasize the importance of performance indicators to monitor health system reform to show how strong primary health care contributes to the realization of universal health coverage.

What is the difference between primary care and primary health care?

A core aspect of primary health care is that it operates in the local community and seeks to address all health problems of all people.[4,9,10] Strong primary health care relies on easy and convenient access to a trusted provider or team of providers. The term "primary care" usually refers to a focus on the health problems of an individual.[1,4,11] Primary health care encompasses a wider

KEY POINTS

- Primary health care addresses the health needs of all patients at the community level, integrating care, prevention, promotion and education.
- Primary health care improves the performance of health systems by lowering overall health care expenditure while improving population health and access.
- The aims of primary health care overlap with those of universal health coverage, which aims to ensure access to essential health services and safe, effective and affordable essential medicines and vaccines for all people.
- To achieve universal health coverage, reforms should focus on strengthening primary health care to ensure equity and cost containment.
- Health system reforms should be monitored with indicators that reflect the core characteristics of primary health care: continuity of care, person- and population-centredness, coordination of care, prevention, health promotion and patient autonomy.

population focus. The distinction between the two is not clear-cut because both terms imply a strong emphasis on prevention, health promotion, education and support delivered in a comprehensive manner. In countries with historically strong primary care, such as the United Kingdom, Denmark and the Netherlands,[12] what is referred to as primary care has broadened in recent decades. Single-physician family practices have shifted to a model of multidisciplinary teams with shared responsibility for the care of target populations. Investment in primary health care in these countries has resulted in more care provided at the community level, and has improved integration of primary care with public health, specialist- and hospital-based care. Thus, the distinction between primary care and primary health care has been blurred. Emphasizing primary health care's focus on the individual is important, because people with seemingly identical health problems may have distinctly different needs,[13] which may become increasingly complex if a patient has multiple chronic health problems.[14]

What is the impact of robust systems of primary health care?

Since the 1978 Declaration of Alma-Ata,[15] which was reinforced by further resolutions of the World Health Assembly,[16] the WHO has promoted primary health care as a core component of health systems.[1] International comparisons of individual countries' performance in population health in relation to their health expenditure and aspects of health care processes and structures have helped us to understand the benefits of effective and efficient primary health care. Starfield's landmark publication in 1994,[12] followed by research from Europe, Canada, the United States and other high-, low- and middle-income countries, has confirmed that health systems with strong primary health care at their core have lower health costs, better population health, higher patient satisfaction, fewer unnecessary hospital admissions and greater socioeconomic equity.[17-20] In addition, these systems have better rates of screening and follow-up for important diseases and are better at addressing the needs of patients with multimorbidity.[21]

How can strong primary health care be achieved?

Strengthening primary health care represents a fundamental shift from health care delivery focused on treating disease toward health systems that address the specific health needs of patients and communities, with a predominant focus on generalism, comprehensiveness and continuity of care (Box 1).[1,4,22] No one size fits all. The process must account for the historical, social, cultural and economic features that shape a country's health system. Primary health care also represents a shift from supply-driven to needs-driven care, toward person-centred support to patients facing the challenges of everyday life, and to people-centred support of communities to strengthen social cohesion and encourage greater resilience.[9,23] Inherent in strong primary health care is reduced reliance on professional care by supporting people to develop and maintain autonomy and to take responsibility for aspects of their own health.

Box 1: Criteria that must be fulfilled to strengthen primary health care[1,22]

- Care provided must be comprehensive (i.e., address all health problems in all patients at all stages of life) and continuous over time.
- Care must be accessible in the local community.
- Gate keepers and coordinators are needed to assist patient referral, when needed, to other health care providers and services.
- Patients should be registered with an individual provider or practice, allowing care to be provided to an identified population of patients over time.
- Training must be based predominantly in primary care settings.
- Health policy support, including equitable payment of primary health care providers compared with their colleagues working in hospitals or in other areas of specialization, is required.

It is important to note that not every country with a strong system of primary health care realizes all of its benefits. For example, only some countries judged to have strong primary health care realized greater efficiency of health care through avoidance of unnecessary hospital admissions and clinical interventions.[19] Political and cultural context in individual countries may affect the overall cohesion and integration of health service functions and thereby affect the implementation of policy.

Much attention has been paid to the relationship of strong primary health care to a nation's total health expenditure. Although health systems research done at the end of last century[12,17,18] reported lower costs in countries with stronger primary health care, more recent European studies have not been able to replicate this finding.[19] However, countries with strong primary health care, such as the UK and the Netherlands, may have invested more in their health systems in recent years, after long periods of limited expenditure in the 1980s and 1990s. We contend that this finding is more a result of national policies of savings and investments rather than the performance of primary health care. Reviewing developments over time with sophisticated indicators to allow comparison between health systems in different countries is important.

A limitation of international comparison studies is the quality of available data, particularly information about primary health care structures and performance. As a consequence, reliable data from well-researched countries like Canada, the UK, Denmark and the Netherlands could dominate the results at the expense of data from countries going through recent system reforms, but where investment in research may be lacking. Standardization of data and the on-going use of data in the monitoring of primary health care policy, as proposed by the Primary Health Care Performance Initiative of the World Bank, the Bill and Melinda Gates Foundation and WHO,[8] should provide more robust information for comparisons between all countries, including low- and middle-income countries.

How can strong primary health care help with realizing universal health coverage?

To achieve universal health coverage, three objectives must be met: everyone — including the poor and patients with the greatest health needs — must have access to care; the health care must be of good quality; and accessing health care should not be prevented by financial barriers. Universal health coverage is expected to increase the use of health care facilities by members of lower socioeconomic groups, which might be expected to increase health care expenditure in the short to medium term, given that people with high unmet health needs will begin to access care.[24,25] Anticipating spending increases could deter governments from making the investment required to achieve universal health coverage, which is why health care reform needs to be understood and committed to over the long term, with a particular focus on strengthening primary health care. Strong primary health care will improve population health through integration of primary care services with public health, thus lowering overall health care expenditure over time, improving the performance of the health care system and ensuring the provision of improved equity and access for everyone.[9] The improved efficiency and cost-effectiveness of care are found in enduring and substantial savings in other parts of health care provision. This result is expected in all countries but is particularly important in low- and middle-income countries with limited resources and economic constraints. Healthier populations[18,19] develop more resilient and socioeconomically viable communities[23,24] that in turn increase the resources available to invest in future services, including health care for all. This is why primary health care should be regarded as a core component in realizing the ambitions of universal coverage as a sustainable development.[2,6,7]

What is the best way to achieve universal health coverage by strengthening primary health care?

Implementation of primary health care and universal health coverage has to take place under prevailing conditions; as a consequence, approaches will differ between countries. Financial demands from previous investments in hospitals and specialist services in many countries may hamper the reallocation of funds within health budgets to primary health care, which can be particularly problematic for low- and middle-income countries.[22] Health policy in many nations is often restricted to the publicly funded health sector, although much health care may be provided privately[22,26] and outside the influence of government-led policies. For example, India has to cope not only with limited health resources for its vast population, but with considerable societal resistance to the principle of health insurance.[26]

Solutions must fit the local socioeconomic and political situation. The UK introduced, and later abolished, fund holding[27] and a quality and outcome framework[28] for primary care, approaches that Denmark and the Netherlands, with similar health care systems, have not implemented. Although the role of the public sector is becoming more prominent in health care in the Netherlands, the country has moved to private health insurance while managing to contain health expenditure.[29] Canadian primary health care has seen the recent introduction of innovations such as greater support for interprofessional primary health care teams, greater adoption of electronic medical records, a strong focus on quality improvement in family medicine[30,31] and greater focus on the management of complex health needs through the pan-Canadian SPOR (Strategy for Patient-Oriented Research) Network in Primary and Integrated Health Care Innovations.[32] International comparisons of primary health care reforms aim to understand the general principles adopted, and the lessons that can be learned from changes taking place under prevailing conditions in each country. However, there is no single ideal set of interventions.

In seeking to attain universal health coverage, the development of sustainable primary health care should continue to be the health policy priority of every nation.[1,3] Implementation of primary health care should be supported by research to improve understanding of how, and to what extent, strengthening it can be done under the prevailing socioeconomic and cultural conditions of the country, and how these conditions will affect the likely costs and efficiency

of future health care provision.[8] To show the effect of investments in primary health care, the success of implementation of interconnected reforms in health systems must be monitored. Indicators need to be developed and applied[4,33] that show the contributions of primary health care (Box 2) and capture characteristics such as continuity of care, person- and population-centredness, coordination of care between health sectors, prevention, health promotion and support for patient autonomy, and a mechanism for data collection must be established. Monitoring these contributions[8] will assist policy-makers to appreciate the contributions made by primary health care toward the attainment of universal health coverage, and support the ongoing investments needed to strengthen and reinforce strong primary health care.

Box 2: Indicators of primary health care[4,33]

- Geographic spread, availability and accessibility of primary health care facilities for patients and communities, with special emphasis on
  - people living in rural and remote locations
  - vulnerable and marginalized groups
- Ability of patients to identify their personal primary health care providers
- Ability of providers to define the population they serve
- Multidisciplinary composition of primary health care services
- Role of primary health care professionals in coordinating all health problems, including
  - acting as gatekeepers for referral to more specialized services and facilities
  - involvement in follow-up and on-going care
- Integration of mental health into primary health care
- Collaboration with other health and support service providers in the community to promote health and well-being of all people
- Equitable income for professionals working in primary health care compared with those working in hospitals and other areas of specialty care
- Training of providers in community settings

References

1. The World Health Report 2008 — primary health care (now more than ever). Geneva: World Health Organization; 2008. Available: www.who.int/whr/2008/en/ (accessed 2017 May 1).
2. Universal health coverage. Sustainable Developmental Goal 3: Health. Geneva: World Health Organization; 2017. Available: http://www.who.int/universal_health_coverage/en/ (accessed 2017 May 1).
3. Sustainable development goals: 17 goals to transform our world. Geneva: United Nations; 2015. Available: www.un.org/sustainabledevelopment/sustainable-development-goals/ (accessed 2017 May 1).
4. Kidd M, editor. *The contribution of family medicine to improving health systems: a guidebook from the World Organization of family doctors*. 2nd ed. London (UK), New York: Radcliffe Publishing; 2013.
5. Jha A, Godlee F, Abbasi K. Delivering on the promise of universal health coverage. *BMJ* 2016;353:i2216.
6. Stigler FL, Macinko J, Pettigrew LM, et al. No universal health coverage without primary health care. *Lancet* 2016;387:1811.
7. Consideration of the recommendations on strengthening community-based health-care services — SEA/RC68/17. New Delhi (India): World Health Organization Regional Office for South-East Asia; 2015.
8. Measuring PHC: the measurement gap. Primary Health Care Performance Initiative; 2015. Available: phcperformanceinitiative.org/about-us/measuring-phc (accessed 2017 May 1).

ANALYSIS

9. Art B, De Roo L, De Maeseneer J. Towards unity for health utilising community-oriented primary care in education and practice. *Educ Health (Abingdon)* 2007;20:74.

10. *The European definition of general practice/family medicine.* Ljubljana (Slovenia): WONCA Europe Secretariat, Institute for Development of Family Medicine; 2011. Available: www.woncaeurope.org/sites/default/files/documents/Definition%203rd%20ed%202011%20with%20revised%20wonca%20tree.pdf (accessed 2017 May 1).

11. Institute of Medicine. *Primary care: America's health in a new era.* Washington: National Academy Press; 1996.

12. Starfield B. Is primary care essential? *Lancet* 1994;344:1129-33.

13. olde Hartman TC, van Ravesteijn H, Lucassen P, et al. Why the "reason for encounter" should be incorporated in the analysis of outcome of care. *Br J Gen Pract* 2011;61:e839-41.

14. Barnett K, Mercer SW, Norbury M, et al. Epidemiology of multimorbidity and implications for health care, research, and medical education: a cross-sectional study. *Lancet* 2012;380:37-43.

15. Declaration of Alma-Alta. *Proceedings of the International Conference on Primary Health Care;* 1978 Sept. 6–12; Alma-Alta, USSR. Geneva: World Health Organization. Available: www.who.int/publications/almaata_declaration_en.pdf (accessed 2017 May 1).

16. Primary health care, including health system strengthening. *Proceedings of the sixty-second World Health Assembly.* Resolution WHA62.12; 2009 May 22. Geneva: World Health Organization. Available: http://www.who.int/hrh/resources/A62_12_EN.pdf (accessed 2017 Oct. 24).

17. Starfield B, Shi L, Macinko J. Contribution of primary care to health systems and health. *Milbank Q* 2005;83:457-502.

18. Macinko J, Starfield B, Shi L. The contribution of primary care systems to health outcomes within Organization for Economic Cooperation and Development (OECD) countries, 1970–1998. *Health Serv Res* 2003;38:831-65.

19. Kringos D. *The strength of primary care in Europe* [thesis]. Utrecht (The Netherlands): Nivel; 2012. Available: www.nivel.nl/sites/default/files/bestanden/Proefschrift-Dionne-Kringos-The-strength-of-primary-care.pdf (accessed 2017 May 1).

20. Schäfer WLA. *Primary care in 34 countries: perspectives of general practitioners and their patients* [thesis]. Utrecht (The Netherlands): Nivel; 2016. Available: www.nivel.nl/sites/default/files/bestanden/w-schafer-pc34.pdf (accessed May 1, 2017).

21. Stange KC, Ferrer RL. The paradox of primary care. *Ann Fam Med* 2009;7:293-9.

22. van Weel C, Kassai R. Expanding primary care in South and East Asia. *BMJ* 2017;356:j634.

23. De Maeseneer J, van Weel C, Daeren L, et al. From "patient" to "person" to "people": the need for integrated, people centered health care. *Int J Pers Cent Med* 2012;2:601-14.

24. De Maeseneer J, Willems S, De Sutter A, et al. *Primary health care as a strategy for achieving equitable care: a literature review commissioned by the Health systems Knowledge Network.* Geneva: World Health Organization; 2007. www.who.int/social_determinants/resources/csdh_media/primary_health_care_2007_en.pdf?ua=1 (accessed 2016 May 1).

25. Watt G. The inverse care law today. *Lancet* 2002;360:252-4.

26. van Weel C, Kassai R, Qidwai W, et al. Primary healthcare policy implementation in South Asia. *BMJ Glob Health* 2016;1:e000057.

27. Kay A. The abolition of the GP fundholding scheme: a lesson in evidence-based policy making. *Br J Gen Pract* 2002;52:141-4.

28. Roland M, Guthrie B. Quality and outcomes framework: what have we learnt? *BMJ* 2016;354:i4060.

29. Kroneman M, Boerma W, van den Berg M, et al. The Netherlands: health system review. *Health Syst Transit* 2016;18:1-240.

30. Hutchison B, Levesque J-F, Strumpf E, et al. Primary health care in Canada: systems in motion. *Milbank Q* 2011;89:256-88.

31. Hutchison B, Glazier R. Ontario's primary care reforms have transformed the local care landscape, but a plan is needed for ongoing improvement. *Health Aff (Millwood)* 2013;32:695-703.

32. Pan-Canadian SPOR Network in Primary and Integrated Health Care Innovations. Ottawa: Canadian Institutes of Health Research; 2017 (modified). Available: www.cihr-irsc.gc.ca/e/49554.html (accessed 2017 Oct. 24).

33. Pettigrew LM, De Maeseneer J, Anderson MI, et al. Primary health care and the Sustainable Development Goals. *Lancet* 2015;386:2119-21.

Competing interests: None declared.

This article was solicited and has been peer reviewed.

Affiliations: Department of Primary and Community Care (van Weel), Radboud University Medical Center, Nijmegen, The Netherlands; Department of Health Services Research and Policy (van Weel), Australian National University, Acton, Australia; Department of Family and Community Medicine (Kidd), University of Toronto, Toronto, Ont.; Murdoch Childrens Research Institute (Kidd), Melbourne, Australia; Southgate Institute for Health, Equity and Society (Kidd), Flinders University, Adelaide, Australia

Contributors: Chris van Weel developed the concept outline of the paper, wrote the first concept of the paper and drafted the final version of the paper. Michael Kidd commented and redrafted the concept outline, commented and redrafted the concept version of the paper and approved its final version.

Correspondence to: Chris van Weel, chris.vanweel@radboudumc.nl

Attribution

Weel C van, Kidd MR. Why strengthening primary health care is essential to achieving universal health coverage. *CMAJ* 2018 April 16;190:E463–466. doi: 10.1503/cmaj.170784. Reproduced with permission.

PART V

CONCLUSIONS

CHAPTER 19

What have we learned and what are the next priorities?

Amanda Howe, Felicity Goodyear-Smith and Chris van Weel

This book presents a snapshot of primary health care development around the globe and highlights common challenges that are encountered. It confirms that health reforms and capacity building of primary health care are taking place in all regions of the world. It stresses that the journey towards primary health care in many countries is in its early days, and will continue over the coming years. As a consequence, the experience we present is directed towards the processes of primary health care reforms – the journey – more than its final destination. This book demonstrates the usefulness of international comparisons in supporting the 'bottom-up' development process of primary health care: applying general values and principles under local socio-economic, political and health system conditions. Experiences from other jurisdictions will hardly ever be implementable on a one-to-one basis; they need to be redesigned to fit the local context. Critical appraisal of experiences from elsewhere, through comparative studies, can help us gain a deeper understanding of the nature of primary health care.

Health reforms aim to find a better fit between the health needs of populations and the care provided, and they should be seen as a continuous, rather than a one-off, process. Populations and their health needs of today may not be the same in the future, and this stresses the importance of an ongoing process of adaptation of health care towards emerging needs – a process that can be informed by comparative studies.

At the same time, the experiences highlight common challenges. Most authors identified patchy policies towards primary health care: for example, specialty training in the primary health care setting being introduced and professional competencies improved but health system regulations still allowing every practitioner to practice in primary health care. Or health system regulations that insufficiently supported the ability of primary health care professionals to apply the skills for which they had been trained. Health reforms should be an integral approach of capacity building through education, training, research and professional development, combined with health system regulations that support the application of the required skills – a comprehensive policy that connects the various policy dots.

To support an integrated policy, measuring the functioning of health systems in terms of primary health care sensitive indicators is a priority. This should include information about continuity of care, integration of mental, physical and social health problems, combining prevention, cure and care, person- and population-centredness, working in a relationship of trust over time, and not being confined to indicators of disease-specific diagnostic and management interventions [1].

A strong academic primary health care infrastructure and leadership is needed to influence policy – at global, regional and local levels [2]. This stresses the importance of 'national' colleges and academies. Primary health care professionals have the best understanding of the complexity of primary health care and its implications for health reforms. What they often forget is how limited the understanding of policy makers is about this complexity. This strengthens the evidence of primary health care – of *what* it contributes to population health, and in particular *how*, through which mechanisms, this is achieved. This is an absolute priority.

Directly related to this come two other priorities on which to focus comparative studies in the coming years. First, the pursuit of universal health coverage [3], and second, gain a better understanding of how to align primary health care and public health at the community level. In this respect, further insight into the functioning of the multidisciplinary primary health care team in the community setting, and in interaction with welfare services, will be of great value.

REFERENCES

1. Primary Health Care Performance Initiative (PHCPI). *Measuring PHC: The measurement gap.* Retrieved from: http://phcperformanceinitiative.org/about-us/measuring-phc (accessed May 1, 2017).
2. Kidd M (editor). *The Contribution of Family Medicine to Improving Health Systems: A Guidebook from the World Organization of Family Doctors.* 2013. Radcliffe Publishing: London, UK (2nd edition).
3. World Health Organization (WHO). *Universal health coverage.* Retrieved from: http://www.who.int/universal_health_coverage/en/ (accessed May 1, 2017).

Index